THE SPIRAL IN THE MAZE

REVEALING A COVER UP OF THE MOST LETHAL PANDEMIC IN HISTORY AND THE SINGLE CAUSE OF MANY DISEASES

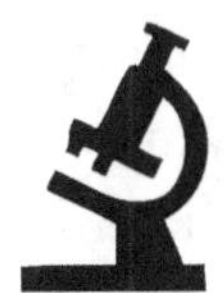

joanna phillips

The Spiral in the Maze by Joanna Phillips

Contributors: Cover design and interior by AuthorPackages.com

ISBN: 9798669925222

Contents

Large Print Version Contents

"When hearing something unusual, do not pre-emptively reject it, for that would be folly. Indeed, horrible things may be true, and familiar and praised things may prove to be lies."

-Ibn Al-Nafis, 13th century physician and researcher who discovered cure for some diseases.

PANDEMICS

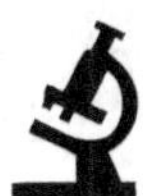

THE GREATEST THREAT TO HUMAN HEALTH - a contagium with rates of mortality and morbidity many times higher than any other pathogen, ever circulating in a continuous pandemic – exists, but the identity of that threat has been covered- up, and death and many diseases have been attributed to 'other' or 'unknown' causes. Some perspective and the degree of threat posed by such a contagium can be realised by looking at the effects of past pandemics.

The 'Spanish' 'flu pandemic of 1918-19 infected an estimated 400 million people (a quarter of the then world population) and, with a mortality rate of about 15%, was responsible for the deaths of between 50 – 100 million. Small pox, with an estimated mortality rate of 30% killed an estimated 500 million in its existence. HIV / AIDS caused more than 36 million deaths at a peak rate of 2 million a year. The Asian 'flu pandemic of 1957-58 killed between 1 and 2 million people. SARS–CoV, causing Severe Acute Respiratory Syndrome in 2002–3, had a relatively high rate of mortality (10%) but only a low rate of infectivity so was only fatal to relatively few, and localized epidemics were contained by actions which slowed down or broke the chain of transmission. However, that virus was not eradicated and, with mutation, was forecast to cause a more lethal and widespread pandemic in the future. The current coronavirus (SARS–CoV–2) pandemic, causing Covid–19, - with a very high rate of transmission and infectivity and a relatively low mortality rate (2-4%?) - has the potential to kill millions worldwide. If a significant percentage of the world population is infected with a pathogen of only a moderate mortality rate, the total number of deaths would be high. It is interesting (and alarming) to compare the 'R' value (the spreadability factor or how many people are infected by a single carrier) of the 'Spanish' 'flu virus (R = 2.1) with that of the current coronavirus (pre-lock-down R = 2.5). That would seem to Indicate a pending global disaster. The R factor indicates the rate of infection in a pandemic and means that a contagium with a high value, even with a relatively low mortality rate, can result in a high number of infected individuals and cause panic and severe disruption of social and economic activity. In all the above epidemics and pandemics, the contagium is a virus, but there have also been pathogenic *bacterial* contagions which have proved fatal to many millions of the population. In the 14th century the 'Black Death' (caused by the bacterium Yersinia pestis) killed an estimated 75 – 200 million people worldwide. During the 20th century Mycobacterium tuberculosis caused 100 million deaths (half of those Infected). But there is one contagium which has rates of transmission, infectivity, mortality and morbidity many times higher than any of the contagions (viral or bacterial) mentioned above, the <u>continuing</u> presence of which HAS BEEN COVERED UP FOR DECADES. The presence of a long-time circulating pathogenic contagium was suspected more than three quarters of a century ago and a decision was made NOT to alert the populace. The realization that the cause of many deaths and diseases had been around for decades, even centuries, and could not be stopped or eradicated at that time (and even now), coupled with the thought that revealing the presence of such a threat to Humanity would cause panic and social and economic chaos, compelled the researchers to restrict their findings to as few people as possible. Thereafter, the collusion, conspiracy and cover-up must have involved members of the medical profession, editing boards of medical journals, governments, the pharmaceutical industry, and the media. Members of the Nobel Prize committee would join that Cabal later. It is plausible that the Hippocratic Oath – 2000 years old but amended many times according to changes in medicine, ethics, attitudes, etc. - has been amended to maintain a veil of secrecy over cover-ups. The more recent amendments promise: *"And whatsoever I shall see or hear in the cause of my profession, as well as outside my profession, in my intercourse with Men, if it be what should not be published abroad, I will never divulge – holding such things to be holy secrets"*. And: *"Whatever I may see or hear in the course of treatment in regard to the life of Man, which on no account one must spread abroad. I will keep to myself, holding such things shameful to be spoken about"*. Because of the cover-up and an inability to *globally* treat and eradicate the Infectious agent (decades ago, and now) the contagium of the pandemic has continued to circulate round the globe, continuing to cause death and disease on a massive scale. Circulating for decades, even centuries, this contagium – a bacterium – has indiscriminately infected all age groups, regardless of ethnicity, geography, etc. In the womb, through life, that bacterium, a spirochaete, remains a sinister and unavoidable threat to BILLIONS of people on the planet. And it may have been suspected centuries ago! A quotation attributed to Desiderius Erasmus in 1520 says *"If I were asked which is the most destructive of all diseases, I should unhesitatingly reply it is that which for some years has been ravaging with impunity. What contagium does thus invade the whole body, so must resist medical art, becomes inoculated so readily, and so cruelly tortures the patient?"*. He asked the question against a background of a mysterious epidemic, hitherto unknown, which struck terror into all hearts by the rapidity of its spread, the ravages it made, and the apparent helplessness of physicians to cure it.

PROSPECTIVE STUDIES

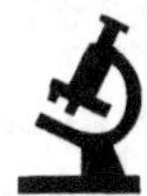

A NUMBER OF STUDIES have been conducted to observe the progress of untreated disease. Common among them for observation was the bacterium Treponema pallidum (Tp) - recognised as the causative organism of syphilis (S). In 1928, a Norwegian retrospective study carried out on several hundred white males, reported on the pathological manifestations of untreated syphilis. Four years later, an American study group decided to build on that Oslo work and perform a <u>prospective</u> study to complement it. [A prospective, observational study is normally employed to look at the long term sequalae of a known or suspected cause, or the effect of suspected risk factors that cannot be controlled. Such epidemiological studies, being observational in nature, examine the causes and development of disease in the human population. Cohorts of subjects are followed over time in longitudinal studies, the population of interest being monitored before, and when, particular disease-related outcomes occur. The studies watch for outcomes such as the development of a disease during the study period, and relate that to factors such as suspected cause or risk.] The American study, conducted between 1932 and 1972 in Tuskegee, Alabama by the US Public Health Service became the infamous and unethical 'Study of untreated syphilis(S) in the negro male' - later to be cited as "arguably the most infamous biomedical research study in US history" and described by one researcher as "the economic exploitation of humans as a natural resource of a disease that could not be cultivated elsewhere, in order to establish and sustain US superiority in patented biotechnology". The Tuskegee Study, the purpose of which was supposedly to observe the natural history of untreated S, was carried out on 600 African-American men who were 'recruited' by being told that they were receiving free health care from the US Government. Two-thirds of the men had previously contracted S before the study began but none were told they had the disease. By 1947, Penicillin had become the standard treatment for (early) S in the general population (and other antibiotics were available in later years), so the doctors involved in the study had the chance of treating all their syphilitic subjects and closing the study, or splitting off a control group for testing with Penicillin . Instead, the Tuskegee researchers continued the study without treating any participants, with-holding the antibiotic and information about it from the men and preventing them from accessing S-treatment programmes in the surrounding areas. The study continued under the control of numerous US Public Health Service supervisors, including the Centre for Disease Control who, in the 1960s reaffirmed the need to continue the study. It ended in 1972 after 40 years of study, when a 'leak' to the media resulted in the trial's termination – the Washington Star, then the New York Times front page article, captured national attention and protest. By the end of the study most of the participants had died from the disease or related complications, 40 wives had been infected and 19 of their children were born with congenital S. The range of mortality and morbidity, and range of complications and disease observed in the 40 years of study, mirrored that of the general population, then and now. The Tuskegee Study, in recognising the threat of Tp to individuals, also revealed the 'credentials' of Tp to be responsible for, and cause, many diseases as it's sequalae. However, that Tp was the single cause of many diseases of the Western world would also remain a secret – known only to the study team and the Cabal of medics, government officials, members of big pharma, and the media, that the team deigned to include in that knowledge. The scale and spread of the disease would, from that time, be masked by censorship. Scientific advisory groups around the world advise and guide governments on health emergencies, but their identity, 'credentials' and work, is shrouded in secrecy so it has always been difficult to challenge the decisions and recommendations being made. Governments do not publish member's names, or their medical or research backgrounds for 'security reasons' and thereby the anonymity of members of the Cabal is maintaIned.

In 1997, President Bill Clinton formally apologised on behalf of the US, to victims of the experiment. The lack of ethical standards in the Study led to the establishment of the Office for Human Research Protections and new federal laws and regulations requiring Institutional Review Boards for the protection of human subjects in studies involving them, but the conclusions of the Study remained unreported. So why the notion and need for a non-treatment experiment? Probably because the researchers knew that S could not be treated on a global scale and eradicated, so needed to observe the natural progression of the disease to determine all of its sequalae.

Other studies had been conducted as the threat of Tp infection to the population was suspected or recognised. In a 1946-47 study in Guatemala, US researchers used prostitutes to infect prison inmates, insane asylum inmates and soldiers with S in order to test the effectiveness of Penicillin as treatment. People who had been infected with direct inoculations of preparations of Tp were also included in the trial. Approximately 700 people, including orphan children, were infected as part of the study which was sponsored by the Public Health Service, the National Institute of Health and the Pan-American Health

Sanitary Bureau (now part of The World Health Organization). The American leader of the team had chosen to do the study in Guatemala because he would not have been permitted to conduct it in the US. He later participated in the Tuskegee Experiment.

THE THEORY OF SINGLE CAUSE

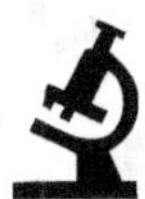

THE SUSPICION THAT A treponeme, as the primary cause of massive mortality and morbidity in the world, carried on a continuously circulating global pandemic and causing many of the major chronic diseases of the human population, is further strengthened by a number of summary premises:

- Tp is a highly infectious bacterium transmissible by virtually every route.

- Tp is not a self-limiting infection, nor is it susceptible to the body's defence mechanisms.

- Tp has been globally widespread for centuries.

- A global programme to eradicate the bacterium has never been implemented.

Given those 4 premises, Tp MUST have spread, and be still spreading, virtually unchecked, resulting in frequent epidemics and global pandemic which will have left the disease endemic in many countries.

Further:

- Tp is known to cause all the clinical sequalae characteristic of many chronic diseases.

- Recognition of S – particularly it's secondary and later manifestations – is difficult.

- Screening for S is limited and the sensitivity of tests for Tp is questionable.

- Administration of anti-Tp antibiotics in high dose, extended course regimens has been very limited, so that most of the global population remains untreated for Tp infection.

The indication is therefore, that many diseases are the result of a single cause – infection by the same contagium (Tp) - which, as main primary cause, satisfies the aetiological, pathological, immunological and epidemiological features and pathogenesis of many diseases. To accept that indication – that a specific disease is caused by a specific organism – the organism should satisfy the basic scientific requirements of 'The Postulates of Koch', which states that:

- The micro-organism must be found in abundance in all subjects suffering from the disease, but should not be found in healthy people.

- The micro-organism must be isolated from a diseased host and grown in pure culture medium.

- The cultured micro-organism should cause disease when introduced into a healthy subject.

- The micro-organism must be re-isolated from the inoculated, diseased, experimental host and identified as being identical to the original, specific, causative agent.

Apart from the inherent limitations that could not be resolved in the late 19th century, and the subtlety and denial of Tp causing many diseases, those postulates do not account for 'agents' that cannot be grown in culture media. Whilst many bacterial pathogens of humans satisfy Koch's postulates, Tp cannot be grown in cell-free culture media, as is also the case for Helicobacter pylori (see later as supposed cause of duodenal ulcer) and the leprosy causing bacterium. They, similarly, do not fulfil all of Koch's postulates.

As previously stated, epidemiologists refer to the *Reproduction Number* (R) which is the number of new infections an infectious person would be able to generate. (common 'flu has a value of 7; measles ca.15). The R number for Tp infection would be very high based on the duration of time that a person is infectious, the opportunities that person has to spread the organism whilst infectious, the probability that with transmission at least one of those opportunities results in infection, and the average susceptibility of the population to that infection. According to that epidemiologists' formula, a very high R value would indicate that the contagium cannot be contained. That established widespread disease and its cause could not be stopped from spreading would have been recognised in the Tuskegee Study.

At any time, without limitation or eradication, the contagium would continue to infect the global population. Tp is highly transmissible by virtually every route but primarily by physical contact, salival transfer, ingestion, and aerosol transmission (the aerosolisation of the bacterium from normal breathing). Sexual transmission of the organism is incidental to the main spread of the disease. Resulting disease, as apparently wide-ranging as Coronary Heart Disease, Sudden Infant Death Syndrome, Multiple Sclerosis, Myalgic Encephalomyelitis (chronic fatigue syndrome), Peptic Ulcer disease, Dementia (and other neurological diseases), Diabetes, Arthritis and others, are <u>different manifestations of the same disease.</u>

A single cause of those diseases would explain many of the specific pathological, immunological and epidemiological features of many diseases, and the links, inter-relationships and commonly observed associations between many of them, and suggests that vertical transmission of Tp rather than genetic inheritance is the explanation of familial traits for some diseases, and that vertical and horizontal transmission of the organism dictates time of onset and spread pattern of many of those diseases. Natural attenuation (especially during vertical transmission of a disease), change, increased host tolerance and the widespread use of antibiotics for unrelated(?) conditions, has probably resulted in forms of Tp and manifestations of its diseases which do not fit the older, classical forms and descriptions of those diseases, making recognition and diagnosis of a disease even more difficult. The effectiveness of sensitivity tests for Tp and current screening procedure is doubted.

Whilst an individual in the early stages of Tp infection can supposedly be cleared of the contagium, and the development of a disease prevented, by administration of a course of an antibiotic (e.g. penicillin), the difficulty in eradicating the highly transmissible pathogen from the global population is obvious, especially as successfully(?) treated individuals are vulnerable to (re)infection the minute they step back into the community. Recognition of those facts was probably the reason for the Tuskegee Study. Tp has a very high R number and, with current global connectivity facilitating even greater transmission possibilities, means that at that level the contagium cannot be contained. The Tuskegee Study group realised that the Tp pandemic was already out of control in the 1940s! Also, just as age, ethnicity, geography and climate have no influence on the distribution of Tp, neither do they affect the intrinsic transmissibility or infectivity of the organism. At best it can be said that social habit (hygiene, dress, isolation) might reduce the opportunities for transmission, but the potential for transmission of the organism by multiple routes in any population – where Tp is anyway known to be circulating (= endemic) - must remain high. S has been globally widespread for centuries and until recently was recognised as one of the most common and important diseases in the world. The oldest known case from which Tp has been isolated was the mummified remains of a 16th century socialite, and the disease was known to be very common by that time. S was first recognised in epidemic form in Europe, and in the Americas post Columbus, in the 15th century, and in the Renaissance Period was known as the Neapolitan disease. Since then, the problems of aetiology and treatment have engaged the attention of many investigators but the fundamental contributions to present knowledge were all made before 1910! The causal organism was identified in 1905 (Schaudinn and Hoffman); a test was developed in 1906 (Wassermann); and a treatment (arsenic) introduced in 1910 (Ehrlick). Early writings going back to Hippocrates make reference to a disease which was probably S. The disease even warranted a poem by Frascatorius in 1530 and a mention in Shakespeare.

Tp is not a self-limiting infection and is not susceptible to the body's defence mechanisms, as evidenced by the fact that the disease can manifest itself many decades after initial infection. The serious clinical sequalae of the infection develop very slowly and insidiously. A mechanism capable of destroying the treponemes in the blood and tissues during secondary S is not known. (It is not phagocytosis as the treponemes seem able to resist engulfment by leucocytes, and lytic processes involving complement and specific antibody have not been identified). Without specific treatment the disease develops and causes a wide range of serious clinical sequalae. The Oslo and Tuskegee Studies were devised to determine the course of untreated S, and from those and other studies it was commonly thought that about 10% of those infected and untreated develop cardiovascular lesions, 10% neurological lesions, and 15% lesions in other tissues, and that 65% of patients with untreated S did not develop late sequalae of the disease – a strange assumption considering the clinical severity of disease in the other 35%! The evidence suggests that the range of clinical sequalae of untreated S is much wider and encompasses many other diseases and degrees of disease. S is a highly infectious disease especially in its early stages, commonly recognised as the first 2 years. Although S is recognised as a sexually transmitted disease, it is known to be transmissible by virtually every other route and non-venereal S is known. It has been supposed that in developed communities especially, transmission was limited because the disease was thought to be spread almost exclusively by sexual intercourse and little opportunity presented for it to be spread by other forms of direct contact under normal conditions of social life. However, it is known that the source of infection can be extra-genital and in non-venereal S rapid transmission of the delicate treponemes occurs – particularly by mouth. All lesions of primary and secondary S – especially those involving the mucous membranes (for which Tp has a particular predilection) on exposed surfaces – discharge very large numbers of treponemes and constitute large reservoirs of infection and a very great hazard. Such lesions may remain infective for as long as 4-5 years until they heal. Other common extragenital sites known include the lips, tongue, mouth, tonsils, pharynx, eye-lids, fingers, hands and any part of the skin and mucous membranes. Infection has been reported in lesions on the hands of medical and nursing staff dealing with cases of S. Further, endemic non-venereal S is known and is common in some countries. It is known that the treponeme responsible for causing *venereal S* and *endemic non-venereal S* is the same – it is morphologically, immunologically, and serologically IDENTICAL. The two diseases are differentiated only by definition based on considerations of climate, geography, age of onset and route of transmission. Venereal S is acknowledged to have global distribution without climatic, geographic, racial or age barriers, whereas non-venereal S has been subjectively delimited to a childhood disease with limited geographical distribution. Such an age definition would automatically exclude any later manifestations of the disease (involvement of vascular tissues, organs, CNS, etc.) some decades later. The fact that endemic non-venereal S (caused by Tp) exists and can affect 60% of some childhood populations confirms the absolute transmissibility and infectivity of the organism via extra-genital sites. That potential for transmission and infectivity must exist globally. The general incidence, spread and development of untreated S, and the range, degree and subtlety of the disease is much greater than has been traditionally thought because the facts and the observations in the long-term prospective studies have been covered up, so for those 'experts' outside the Cabal, the disease has spread unrecognised, unchecked and mis-diagnosed. A coordinated global programme to eradicate Tp infection has never been implemented. The disease is acknowledged to have been globally widespread for centuries and by the afore-mentioned premises must have continued to spread. An effective treatment for an individual has only been available, or applied, in the last 80 years, and previous epidemics must have left a massive reservoir of untreated, infected (and infectious) individuals. *Recognised* early infectious S reached its peak just after the second world war and the advent of penicillin supposedly made a dramatic and rapid impact on that incidence of disease. Early WHO-orchestrated programmes in parts of Africa, the Middle East and Yugoslavia had limited success, but for a variety of reasons (socio-economic, competing medical priorities, health administrators over-impressed by early success, etc.) such programmes were not properly consolidated, nor further continued, nor expanded into other areas, so that relapse and re-infection resulted. Treatment of whole communities in a national, international or global progamme to eradicate the disease has never been undertaken. That must have left the vast majority of the world population untreated, to constitute a large reservoir of infection with massive potential for continued transmission, so the disease would remain endemic in some countries and a global pandemic would continue. The continuing high prevalence of S in developing countries, and the 'resurgence' of the disease in advanced countries was recognised and noted by the WHO more than 40 years ago.

Although antibiotics have since been widely used for a range of infections, relatively few individuals will have received an appropriate antibiotic in high enough dosage administered at the right time or for long enough time to eradicate Tp so spread of the disease in all infected populations must have continued. Even those few individuals successfully(?) treated would be liable to re-infection as continuous interface, interaction and traffic at family, community, national and international level would facilitate continuous spread of the disease, unless a global policy of effective treatment of the population was undertaken. The risk of an outbreak of S from an individual presenting with classic symptoms of the disease and the threat of Tp infection to any population *is* currently recognised and guarded against. However, current screening policy – that employed in routine diagnosis and mass screening programmes – is heavily reliant on tests designed to indicate disease *activity*. Such tests often react negatively in late or latent disease and will fail to indicate the extent of vertically acquired disease or disease contracted horizontally early in life. What has not been recognised nor guarded against by those outside the Cabal is the absolute transmissibility of the bacterium, the less than classic and wide range of symptoms of later disease and the risk to the global population – factors which demand a coordinated treatment policy on a global scale. Those factors have been covered up (with an admission that an effective treatment was not available for a global population and the pandemic has long been out of control?), so without such a policy the disease has spread, and will continue to spread throughout the global population. It is worth noting that the current and earlier coronavirus infections achieved global distribution in months, and the AIDS virus - with limited routes of transmission and a relatively low rate of infectivity - in less than two decades. By contrast, the potential of an infectious agent which has been around for centuries, is transmissible by virtually all known routes, and has never been 'challenged' globally, must be unlimited. WHO acknowledges 40 million new cases of S being notified worldwide annually. That must be the 'tip of the iceberg'. With the possible exception of small isolated communities, Tp infection must be currently endemic in most countries, and in a continuing pandemic, billions of the world's population must have been infected.

Treponema pallidum is KNOWN to cause all the clinical sequalae shown by, and characteristic of, the major chronic diseases. WHO's *International Classification of Diseases* devotes more pages to, and attributes more clinical sequalae to syphilis than any other disease. It is known that Tp can affect virtually every tissue, organ and system of the body and can cause most conditions and mimic most 'other' diseases. The clinical signs of disease attributed to Tp infection are clinically indistinguishable from the clinical signs attributed to supposed other causes. For example, the signs of cardiovascular disease attributed to Tp are no different from those of aortic incompetence and aneurysms from 'other' causes. S has always been known as the most subtle of all diseases and thought a master of disguise. There is no symptom that it cannot cause, and no syndrome for which it may be responsible. Virtually every disease in part has been attributed to Tp infection. Research, as in the Tuskegee Study and others, suggests that Tp infection is the MAIN cause of those diseases.

Recognition of the disease at any stage is difficult. Any of the stages of the disease can be absent or so inapparent as to be overlooked, and a diagnosis of S from its secondary and later clinical signs would be unlikely. Primary infection with Tp and first clinical signs of S ('flu-like illness, adenitis, etc.,) are often missed, and without that recognition subsequent clinical manifestations of the disease many years later (coronary heart disease, dementia, etc.) will be most unlikely to be diagnosed as S or be associated with that disease. S is a general systemic infection in the course of which certain lesions are produced in different tissues which may be sufficiently striking to attract medical attention. Without recognition of the primary disease, those lesions will almost certainly be labelled 'other disease'. Such manifestations of S will most often be mis-diagnosed. As a result, most such patients will never be tested for S, have their condition diagnosed as S, or be treated for S. As an illustration, a patient presenting with later manifestations of the disease – such as damage to the cardiovascular system with destruction of elastic tissue and formation of aneurysms in the large arteries - would (without recognition of the primary phase) be diagnosed *only* as having coronary heart disease. Recognition of Tp infection in the clinical situation is extremely poor. The Tuskegee Study showed that the incidence of sub-clinical disease (especially cardio-vascular lesions and aortitis) was at least twice as high as clinically diagnosed disease, and there is evidence that patients with S are more prone to 'other' diseases.

Screening for Tp infection in the population is limited. The bacterium is hard to find and identify, and the sensitivity of tests for it is questionable and further compromised by many factors. Essentially, to be diagnosed positive for Tp infection depends on when and how an individual is tested. Confirmation of Tp infection, and diagnosis of S, even for the few showing classical primary clinical signs (as in those with venereal S) is extremely difficult, and standard tests for S - the tests most likely to be employed in general screening procedures - are not sufficiently specific or sensitive for complete diagnostic reliability and results can also be compromised by other factors. It is known that in primary S, none of the tests available is 100% conclusive, even if conducted at the right time relative to the time of initial infection, and ALL serological tests can be negative despite the presence of a primary lesion. Further tests are supposedly more specific but would normally only be carried out if initial screening results were positive and are, anyway, compromised by a number of factors. It is known that the available tests can be variously compromised by lack of specificity; lack of serological reactivity of the bacterium (which may be due to a capsular or slime layer sometimes observed on the surface of Tp); scarcity of treponemes (as in very early, latent and late stages of the disease); slow or non-appearance of antibody (reagin) in serum; excess reagin normally produced in some patients; and antibiotic usage (even months before). All those factors would induce a negative reaction to the tests. Positive reactions can be similarly misleading and can be caused by many (other) microbial infections and pathological lesions (which can liberate lipid antigens in the tissues and consequently form lipoidophil antibodies on which some tests are based). Supposed false positive reactions are frequently seen in blood donors, pregnant women, and those with an infection, but are usually attributed to other factors, or contradicted by further tests. Infections such as glandular fever, mumps, chicken pox, herpes simplex, herpes zoster and viral(?) pneumonia can cause positive results to a test many months after the infection, and rheumatoid arthritis and many auto-immune diseases (disseminated lupus erythematosus, haemolytic anaemia, thyroiditis, etc.) can cause positive reactions to those tests for many years, even a life-time. The fact that rheumatoid arthritis, many supposed auto-immune diseases, microbial infection, and unconfirmed glandular fever and mumps show positive to standard tests for S would seem to confirm the presence of Tp. It is suggested that many of the supposed *false* positive reactions are in fact a *true* positive reaction to Treponema pallidum. The fact that the KNOWN incidence of false positive and false negative results in those tested is high, must question the effectiveness of the screen for Tp – a screen which anyway is reserved for a very small percentage of patients selected from genito-urinary departments, ante-natal clinics, transplant centres, blood transfusion centres and some neurological wards. The sensitivity of available tests and even the premise on which some of them are based (eg: antibody production) is questionable. The presence of Tp, at whatever stage in the progression of the disease, is extremely difficult to determine even by trained analysts, but an inability by Science to show the presence of Tp does not mean that it is not present, or has not been present, as the causative organism of a particular disease. It is known that in Tabes Dorsalis for example (an extreme and advanced form of S) Tp is NOT found in the tissues. Like many bacterial infections the chronicity of the inflammatory reaction is often inversely proportional to the number of organisms seen, and that phenomenon is apparent in the many diseases caused by Tp. In late or latent cases of syphilis ALL tests (even the more specific tests) can be negative, and a high percentage (>20%) of late cases react negatively to the standard tests for S. Also, the fact that even after supposedly adequate treatment with appropriate antibiotics, the VDRL test can remain positive for some time, and the FTA and TPHA tests often remain positive for life. That must seriously question the sensitivity of the tests, or the effectiveness of treatment, or both, or invite the conclusion that Tp is present and that those tests are showing true positives. It must be remembered anyway, that the vast majority of patients suffering secondary and later manifestations of S (such as cardiovascular disease, dementia, MS, arthritis, etc.) will never have been suspected of having S so will not have been subjected to those tests. Being in older age groups with long-standing disease, they would probably test negatively anyway. Even with such limitations, random screening of an aged population will show >2.5% of them to have Tp infection and in those tested for the infection the number of confirmed infected individuals is greatly underestimated. The effectiveness of testing is therefore doubted and supportive claims for the effectiveness of the tests have not enough basis to deflect anything from these facts.

Administration of antibiotics which are active against Tp and which are given at high enough dosage or for long enough time to eradicate the organism is very limited. Unless a patient is being treated specifically for confirmed S, most antibiotics – employed empirically to treat other infections – are unlikely to be given in a regimen effective enough to eradicate Tp, even if the bacterium was included in its spectrum of antibacterial activity. That means that for most of the global population and despite the widespread use of antibiotics, without recognition and correct diagnosis of the primary disease, the secondary and later manifestations of the disease will be un-treated, under-treated or mis-treated.

Procaine penicillin (by injection) remains the treatment of choice for all types of (confirmed) S and successful treatment depends on achieving high blood and tissue concentrations and maintaining those over at least two weeks. 100% cure rates are unknown, and cure rates for other antibiotics in the treatment of S (e.g. oral erythromycin, tetracyclines, cephalosporins) are significantly lower even when used at the required levels, and in empirical use for other infections would be most unlikely to effect clinical cure and eradication of the bacterium. The effectiveness of antibiotic therapy is difficult to determine. Tp is supposedly extremely sensitive to penicillin and during treatment healing of lesions occurs and the treponemes disappear from early stage lesions. Biological cure however (= complete eradication of the treponemes) is difficult to prove since the bacterium cannot be cultured in vitro. It is known that in some patients who have been 'adequately' treated with procaine penicillin, residual treponemes have been detected in cerebro-spinal fluid and lymph nodes. Those bacteria have not acquired resistance to the antibiotic because surviving treponemes, after inoculation into rabbits, produce typical lesions where they are penicillin sensitive. It may be then that the treponemes migrate to less accessible tissues, such as neural and skeletal tissue, where levels of antibiotic are not sufficiently high to effect complete eradication of that bacterial population so that reservoirs of treponemes remain in those tissues. The potential for a large number of infected individuals to remain in any population, even after treatment, therefore must be significant.

The prognosis for treated S depends on the stage of the disease and the degree of tissue damage that has occurred in vascular, neurological and other systems. Whilst successful treatment may result in clinical cure and stop the inflammatory process and progression of disease, the tissue damage may have been too great to prevent an improvement in symptoms and the disease would be regarded as chronic.

The widespread use of antibiotics for unrelated(?) conditions has probably resulted in forms of Tp and manifestations of S which do not fit the older, classical, clinical definitions, which must confuse further the clinical picture and make diagnosis even more difficult. As previously said, such antibiotics, in empirical use, are unlikely to be given in high enough dose or for long enough to eradicate Tp even if they are active against the bacterium. The most widely used antibiotic in the UK – amoxycillin – is not active against Tp in normal dosage regimens. It is interesting to note that in the US and Japan - where cephalosporin antibiotics have been used extensively for the past 20 years - the incidence of coronary heart disease has coincidentally declined. Cephalexin for example is active against Tp if given as high dose, extended courses. It may be then, that the widespread use of certain antibiotics may have had some effect in limiting the progression of Tp infection, but the incidence of late manifestations of the infection would remain high. Such an observation would indicate that a globally implemented antibiotic programme might have some success and benefit future generations, but implementing such a programme would not be possible in practical terms. That was recognised by the Tuskegee Study team and was the reason for the Study.

PATHOLOGY AND PATHOGENESIS

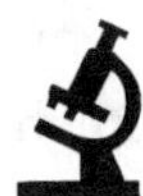

IN LOOKING AT THE pathology and pathogenesis of Tp infection, it is suggested that infection by that bacterium – achieved by virtually any route of transmission to any of a number of sites (mainly mucous membranes of the nasopharynx, mouth and digestive tract) – results in the first clinical signs of penetration such as chancre and ulcer of the mouth, stomach or duodenum. Where the infection occurs 'in utero' (Tp can cross the placental barrier), conditions such as hole in the heart and cleft lip and palate may result. Tp is a spirochaete (a spiral organism), superbly designed for penetration into even intact tissue and capable of boring, corkscrew and thrusting movements. (Also, it is now known that the bacterium is micro-aerophilic rather than a strict anaerobe – a property which facilitates transfer outside the body.) After penetrating tissue, the treponemes invade the perivascular lymph spaces where they multiply rapidly and massively to excite the syphilitic reaction. That consists of an accumulation of mononuclear cells (lymphocytes and monocytes) to form a focus of inflammatory tissue which is highly vascular. Fibroblasts are stimulated to proliferate and 'healing' occurs with replacement of inflammatory cells by fibrous tissue. The degree of fibrosis and the type of host tissue would determine the visibility of the initial chancre or ulcer which can be very discreet, especially in thin mucous membranes. Such lesions, and any serum that exudes from them, contain very large numbers of treponemes and all lesions of secondary S – especially those involving mucous membranes on exposed surfaces – discharge very large numbers of treponemes. As such they constitute large reservoirs of infective material for transmission and a very great hazard. Such lesions may remain infective for as long as 4-5 years, until they heal. A site in the mouth therefore would have a potential for infecting others (by aerosol droplet or salival transfer) and might facilitate a direct route to the central nervous system via the mucous membranes and the sinuses.

Before the first lesion has appeared (commonly 10 – 90 days after initial infection) the treponemes undergo massive multiplication (with a generation time of less than 5 hours are capable of producing billions of organisms in days) and infect the entire body. Initially the treponemes invade the lymph nodes where they cause an adenitis, and from the regional lymphatics are rapidly conveyed to the blood stream in large numbers, and from there to the various tissues. The adenitis at this stage would most likely be diagnosed as 'viral infection', 'glandular fever' or 'mumps' and as such would not be treated. A common clinical sign of Tp infection at this stage is a 'flu-like illness, often severe and of protracted length, which usually occurs within 3 months of initial infection. Tp has a known predilection for mucous membranes and the fact that 'respiratory infection', a 'cold' or 'snuffles' is a common pre-cursor to infant cot death (which commonly occurs around 3 months of age) strongly implicates Tp and infection in the first few days / weeks of life, as the primary cause of Sudden Infant Death Syndrome. A 'flu-like reaction to Tp infection is only one of a number of known initial clinical signs. Other indications of such infection include headaches, swollen glands, rashes, general malaise, iritis and conjunctivitis, gastritis, weight loss, and meningitis. In the very young, the elderly, sick or immuno-compromised, this first manifestation of Tp infection may be fatal. Occasionally, patients can suffer recurring 'first manifestations' with recurrent bouts of colds, 'flu, and throat and respiratory tract infections. Glandular fever or 'recurrent infection' would commonly be diagnosed. After such clinical sequalae which, without notice of a primary syphilitic reaction, would be mis-diagnosed and therefore untreated or mis-treated, the disease can enter a period of quiescence during which time the foci of infection can remain dormant and undetected in the tissues for a long time. Alternatively, the disease develops insidiously to cause later serious clinical sequalae, but whereas early clinical manifestations of S are probably due to the vast numbers of treponemes and their effects, later manifestations of the disease are probably the result of delayed hypersensitivity and inflammatory reactions to the products or toxins of the bacterium and the presence of relatively few persisting treponemes. Like other chronic bacterial infections (e.g. tuberculosis) chronicity of the inflammatory reaction is often inversely proportional to the number of organisms seen, and lesions of tertiary S contain very few treponemes. Over a long period, certainly years, sometimes decades, it is thought that Tp causes a general demyelination of fatty tissues - a destruction of fats and muco-proteins - or an interference with their metabolism, causing breakdown of elastic tissue, extensive tissue damage and exposure of nerve fibres. Such effect may be mediated by immune complexes. A principal pathological effect of Tp infection is damage to the cardiovascular system with destruction of elastic tissue and the formation of aneurysms in the large arteries. Tp is believed to spread to the aorta during the early stages of the infection, possibly via the lymphatics and the mediastinal nodes. The treponemes lodge in the aortic wall and may remain dormant for years. The eventual consequence is destruction of the muscular and elastic layers of the aortic wall and replacement with functionally inert scar tissue. Sudden unexpected death is frequently associated with aortic regurgitation and angina. It is estimated that in those patients with cardiovascular lesions, 30% died as a direct result of it, and lesions of cardiovascular S are not infrequently found at autopsy in selected populations as a chance finding. It has also been observed that simple syphilitic aortitis has been diagnosed in 5 – 10% of people during life.

In the smaller arteries and capillaries, at a more discreet level or earlier in the process, such effect may cause general hypertension or, in the heart, coronary insufficiency. Hyperlipidaemia and atherosclerosis may be the result of deposition of degraded fatty materials leached from tissues, or a compensatory response by the body to make up the 'loss' caused by the effects of Tp infection. Changes in fat composition have also been observed in the liver of victims of SIDS, and in peptic ulcer disease mucous loss is noticeable at the site of ulceration.

In the lung, disease of the small pulmonary arteries would cause pulmonary hypertension with associated symptoms and sequalae. In the brain, the degree of narrowing of the arteries might variously cause headaches, migraine, neuroses, psychoses, epilepsy and dementia before any cerebral atrophy or thrombosis is identified. In Diabetes, carbohydrate and fat metabolism is disordered and the defect leads to the appearance of atherosclerosis early in patients with that disease. Atherosclerosis itself may be a compensatory response by the body (working on negative feedback instruction) to make up the 'loss' caused by Tp.

It has been established that many patients with rheumatoid arthritis die from infections and renal diseases, and in some studies an increased mortality from cardiovascular, gastro-intestinal and respiratory diseases was reported. A reported excess of deaths from malignancies in patients with rheumatoid arthritis remains controversial.

Damage to the CNS remains sub-clinical for a long time – often several decades – but at an extreme would include destruction of the fatty coating around nerve fibres. In some CNS disorders it is known that an accumulation of amyloid precursor protein (APP) causes impairment of axonal transport with deposition of amyloid and plaque formation, and recent studies have shown that axon degeneration precedes and sometimes causes neural death. Dying back processes may underlie early loss of synapses that occurs in Alzheimers disease for example. Other CNS disorders with APP positive axon pathology include the acute demyelinating diseases such as Parkinsonism, MS, Motor Neuron Disease, Creutzfeldt-Jakob disease, senile dementia and HIV dementia. In Alzheimers, MND and Parkinsonism, damage to specific regions of the CNS leaves the affected areas especially prone to the consequences of neuronal attrition. Tp should be considered as one of the 'triggers' and cause of axon death in many disorders.

Different symptoms of the disease are probably a result of the different tissues developing hypersensitivity to Tp and its products and reacting differently to the irritation with different inflammatory responses and degrees of response. The fat and muco-protein loss results in an overall 'drying out' and loss of lubrication and elasticity in the affected tissue which can then become hypersensitive to irritants and liable to dysfunction. Such reaction is classically seen in asthma, hay fever and skin disease such as eczema, which are often related. A greater and chronic inflammatory response is observed in lupus erythematosus and arthritis. Other principal pathological effects include the formation of chronic granulomata in skin, bone, the internal organs and the brain. A dose response relationship would be expected for neuronal damage of infectious origin and there could be considerable interindividual variation in susceptibility. Trace of the causative organism is often gone long before the appearance of those diseases.

Evidence of a direct link between chronic sinusitis and MS (by spread of infection from a diseased sinus into the CNS) once prompted examination of an old 'spirochaetal hypothesis' which has been shown to be not erroneous, and a spirochaetal infection of the CNS would explain the specific pathological, immunological and epidemiological features of MS.

The degree of association between Schizophrenia and organic disease exceeds that expected by chance and it is thought that in some cases the organic disease is of major aetiological importance. The most common organic states associated with Schizophrenia are epilepsy, neurosyphilis, alcohol and drug abuse, and those common associations cannot be dismissed as chance findings as they occur too often in the presentation and course of schizophrenic illness to be ignored. Those observations suggest that most such supposed age-related neuronal attrition is a consequence of demyelination of nerve tissue due to infection by Tp. It is therefore suggested that demyelination is mediated by immune complexes as a result of infection with Tp and that **TREPONEMA PALLIDUM IS THE PRIMARY CAUSE OF A NUMBER OF DISEASES.**

RANGE OF DISEASE

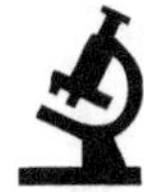

TP INFECTION IS UBIQUITOUS and largely sub-clinical for many years. The initial infection might take place before birth or in very early life although the disease may not appear until much later. The infection can be passed through sperm or the ovum and be transmitted trans-placentally, perinatally or postnatally through close contact. The body's inability to deal with the bacterium would then allow the development of future disease. The diseases include those of the vascular tissues - heart attack, stroke, hypertension, atherosclerosis and hypercholesteraemia and 'cluster meningitis'; diseases of the CNS such as senile and familial transmissible dementia, motor neuron disease, Parkinson's disease and Alzheimer's disease; obstructive airways disease, asthma and recurrent 'bronchitis'; rheumatoid and osteo-arthritis; ME; skin disease including eczema, psoriasis and varicose ulcers; multiple sclerosis; duodenal and gastric ulcer disease; Crohns disease; Sudden Infant Death Syndrome and 'in utero' events such as cleft lip, cleft palate (the world's 3rd most common birth defect), hole in the heart, still-birth and spontaneous abortion. In SIDS, the finding of unusually high levels of immunoglobins in the lungs of cot death babies lends weight to the theory that death results from an anaphylactic reaction to a respiratory infection. Victims of the syndrome often have an upper respiratory tract infection in the week before death so the pathogen would have stimulated or disrupted the immunoglobin production system and exposed the infant to a full attack from the bacterium. Reyes Syndrome is an acute childhood illness with vomiting and coma that typically occurs a few days after a mild infection and the pathogenesis is usually attributed to generalized mitochondrial dysfunction caused by a bacterial, viral or toxic agent in a genetically susceptible host. Crohns disease and ulcerative colitis are ten times more common in immediate family members of patients with those diseases compared with the general population. A link between a bacterium and Crohns disease has not been clearly established but controlled trials have shown that long-term treatment with an antibiotic (metronidazole, effective against anaerobes) can be effective in both colonic and peri-anal Crohns disease. Investigations to determine whether an infectious agent is involved in the aetiology of Crohns suggest that because the occurrence of the disease in married couples is greater than that expected by chance, spouses of patients might be at particular risk of contracting the disease, which supports the view that an infectious agent might be involved. Most of those diseases are KNOWN as late manifestations of Tp infection and catalogued as such in the WHO 'Classification of Diseases'. It is worth noting that 'an infectious agent' or 'unknown virus *infection*' is often proposed in the aetiology of many of those diseases. Newspaper headlines many years ago posed the question "is infection the cause of a heart disease epidemic?"

Recognising Tp as the primary cause of many diseases also explains the commonly observed associations, links and inter-relationships of many supposed 'distinct' diseases. Such associations are known between asthma and eczema, hypertension and obstructive airways disease, diabetes and skin disease, retinopathy and blindness, osteomyelitis and cutaneous chronic ulcers, sinusitis and MS, and sexually transmitted disease and 'juvenile' arthritis. Also, as an objective overview, this hypothesis unifies many diseases which are currently only differentiated by subjective interpretation, description and name. Similarly, it offers an alternative explanation to genetic inheritance for some diseases. Vertical transmission of Tp would account for familial traits seen in coronary heart disease, hypertension, atherosclerosis, hypercholesteraemia, asthma, eczema, ulcerative colitis, Crohns disease and some dementias. Early, juvenile and late onset forms of many diseases would be a result of the time of initial Infection with Tp relative to either vertical or horizontal transmission of the organism - as where traditional adult diseases occur in children (stroke in infants; heart attack in juveniles). The organism can cross the placental barrier and can be transmitted to the foetus throughout pregnancy. The degree of maternal disease *activity* probably dictates the time of onset and severity of disease in pregnancy, so that the effect may range from extreme and immediate (intra-uterine or neonatal death) through congenital disease in the infant or child, to more subtly manifest disease many years later in the adult. Second and third generation S is known. Vertically acquired infection may also render the individual refractory to subsequent horizontal infection. Additional support for this thinking comes from the fact that treponemes have actually been identified in association with some diseases (peptic ulcer disease and multiple sclerosis) and postulated as the cause of MS via the sinuses. In the early 1900s several reputable neuropathologists noted the similarity of the clinical and histological characteristics of MS and neurosyphilis, and reported the presence of treponemes in the plaques of Multiple Sclerosis. **The theory that Multiple Sclerosis was caused by a treponeme has never been disproved.**

In the light of this hypothesis Tp should also be considered as the primary cause of Guillain-Barre disease, Creutzfeldt – Jacob disease, Reiter's syndrome, Henloch-Schlonlein purpura, Gertsmann – Straussler syndrome, Erythema Infectiosum (5th Disease), Occult Subacute Thyroiditis. And Cancer? - Tp might be implicated in the aetiology of lymphomas (Hodgkin's Disease) and leukaemias (see later).

This hypothesis may also offer an explanation for the development of full-blown AIDS after HIV infection. It is thought that other factors besides the virus are needed for a substantial lowering of T4 cell levels and progression to full blown AIDS. Tp itself can profoundly depress T4 cell levels and may be an important contributor or co-factor. Seroconversion studies have suggested that sexually transmitted co—factors, pre-seroconversion and/or post-seroconversion, play a role in the progression of HIV infection. The effect may simply be additive when the rate of progression from HIV infection to full-blown AIDS would be dictated by the degree of syphilitic <u>activity</u> in the presence of the virus. Fastest actual decline could be anticipated if Tp infection or early active disease occurred at the time of HIV infection or sometime post-seroconversion (Tp acting on the viral genes that regulate HIV expression in the host cell); slowest decline could be anticipated if the virus infection occurred on top of a late or latent syphilitic state, or if Tp was not present. Where latent S exists, destruction of the immune system by HIV might allow development of a disease in the same way as latent TB develops when 'unmasked' by the virus. Alternatively, HIV might act purely opportunistically in a Tp compromised host, or similarly Tp in an HIV compromised host. Widespread incidence of Tp infection would explain the ultimate high conversion rate of HIV infection into full-blown AIDS. In all those scenarios, appropriate antibiotic treatment and long-term prophylaxis might mean HIV infection not progressing to full-blown AIDS.

DIVERSIONARY MEASURES

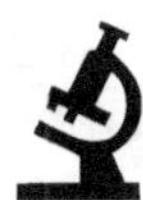

T HERE HAVE BEEN MANY outbreaks of disease which could be attributed to Tp as the cause, and some diseases and cause appear to have been deliberately covered up, viz: The Tuskegee study and Helicobacter pylori causing ulcers study. In the early 1980s a physician at the University of Western Australia, set out to show that the bacterium Helicobacter pylori (Hp) played a major role in causing peptic ulcer disease, challenging decades of medical doctrine holding that ulcers were caused primarily by stress, spicy foods, excess acid, etc., and instead adopted the theory that peptic ulcers were caused by a bacterium – an idea first postulated 150 years ago (Bottcher and Letulle, 1875). The presence of bacteria-like organisms in the lumen of the gastric glands was also noted by Klebs in 1881, and Jaworski in 1889 described spiral organisms in sediment washings of humans and suggested those organisms might be involved in gastric ulcer disease. A century ago, different researchers found spirochaetes in the stomachs of mice, cats, dogs and cows, and in the early 20th century a number of researchers found spirochaetes associated with peptic ulcer disease. In 1936, the first edition of the Russian 'Large Medical Encyclopaedia' suggested infection was one of the causes of peptic ulcer disease. In 1939

Friedberg found Hp in the human stomach but abandoned his research after his boss advised him to move to another subject! Hp was generally regarded as a harmless commensal organism in the stomachs of millions of people. In the 1950s a number of researchers (Allende, in 1951, Tarnopolskaya in 1955, Gordon in 1958) used penicillin to treat gastric ulcers, and since then numerous researchers found bacteria associated with peptic ulcer disease. Their reported findings were often rejected for publication.

In 1982 the researchers in Australia began their first study to determine the relationship between Hp and peptic ulcer disease (PUD) The letters referencing that research were published in the Lancet in 1983. A year later, one of the research team intentionally consumed a large inoculum of Hp and became ill (as would be expected with the ingestion of any bacterial culture!) He then self-medicated with antibiotics and was relieved of his symptoms and those observations were published in 1985. **INGESTING THE CULTURE OF Hp DID NOT INDUCE AN ULCER.** Ingestion of Hp has been shown to cause gastritis in many animal subjects but has NEVER been shown to induce ulcer formation. The claim that eradication of the bacterium (in this case Hp) with antibiotics and substantially reducing the occurrence of ulcers would equally apply to any bacterium (including Tp which has better 'credentials' for causing ulcers). Hp is linked aetiologically to histological GASTRITIS but a pathogenic role for Hp in duodenal ulcer (DU) disease is unproven and whilst Hp might fulfil Koch's postulates for histological GASTRITIS, it does not fulfil them for DUODENAL ULCERATION. Studies suggest that eradication of Hp infection is associated with a significant reduction in the relapse rate of DU, independent of other factors. In patients remaining culture negative for one year, both histological gastritis and DU recurrence were unlikely. That does not prove that Hp is of aetiological importance in DU disease. Hp has been implicated in the pathogenesis of gastritis, DUs, GUs and even gastric cancer but ASSOCIATON and CAUSE should not be confused. Hp is a bacterium which characteristically grows attached to gastric epithelial cells and is commonly found in the gobal population with easy transmission (orally or by ingestion), usually within families. That makes it an ideal 'fall-guy' to divert attention from other possible causes. It was observed that patients with recurrence of Hp infection tended to experience relapse of their DU disease, whereas those in whom complete eradication had been achieved were much less likely to have a recurrence of duodenal ulceration. That would be the case if another bacterium was the causal organism. Examination of the distribution of peptic ulcer sites has revealed that they occur most commonly on either side of the pyloric sphincter. In the stomach, ulceration of the gastric mucosa occurs in the narrowed part of the stomach where transition of Tp from a contaminated bolus of food and penetration into the near-by gastric wall would be relatively easy, and a gastric ulcer would result. After exit through the pylorus, a contaminated bolus would immediately enter the narrowest section of the duodenum and the bacterium would be close to the duodenal mucosa with opportunity for transmission from the food bolus and perforation of the duodenal wall to cause a duodenal ulcer.

Evidence that infection precedes the first ulcer is difficult to prove because endoscopy is rarely done in people without symptoms. In DU relapse however, recurrence of Hp infection after apparent eradication is probably due to the original strain surviving antibiotic treatment (indicating failure of eradication), re-infection with Hp or a less sensitive causative bacterium. Pharmaceutical company promotional literature to doctors at that time showed that recurrence of Hp after treating the ulcer with antibiotics was very low. The literature did not show recurrence rates of PUD. An extensive study in Dublin demonstrated that eradication of Hp with antibiotics substantially reduced the re-occurrence of ulcers, but that would also be the result if the antibiotics were eradicating a different causative bacterium. Ingestion of Hp has been shown to cause gastritis in many animal studies (and by the researcher himself!) but has NEVER been shown to induce an ulcer. Nowhere has Hp been shown to be the cause of peptic ulcers; the evidence is only circumstantial. As previously stated, Hp fulfils Koch's postulates for histological gastritis but does not fulfil them for duodenal ulceration, but the researchers' claims got antibiotics used for ulcer treatment, and the recommended regimens would be effective against treponemal infection and true cause. The lead researcher was awarded the Nobel Prize in 2005. But for what? The formulation of a new cocktail? Hp broth as a new gastronomic treat? Certainly not for identifying the cause of PUD. That award questions the gullibility, integrity or involvement with the Cabal of those Stockholm and Frankfurt committees and the committee awarding the Ehrlich and Darmstaedter prize in 1977. The research was continued in the US where the process was required to be accelerated - which ultimately the National Institute of Health and the FDA did by fast-tracking a lot of the existing 'knowledge' into the US, and getting others to conduct repeat studies to *confirm* the results and 'get the news out' (1990s). A conference held by the NIH(USA) demonstrated the general acceptance in the US of Hp as the cause of PUD. The medical community had been finally convinced; the cover-up had been consolidated. Despite the conclusions and claims for Hp, the lead researcher still conceded that an infectious cause for most diseases that remain unexplained could not be ruled out.

CANCER

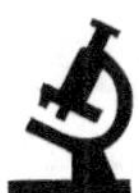

THE RESEARCHER ALSO CLAIMED that Hp was the cause of stomach cancer. He had observed that everybody who got stomach cancer developed it on a background of gastritis, and in patients without Hp, gastritis was not evident. He concluded that because the only important cause of gastritis was Hp (according to him), therefore that bacterium had to be the most important cause of stomach cancer as well!! Treponema pallidum would be a better candidate as the causal agent for stomach cancer (and for other cancers as well). As previously stated, that researcher had conceded that many diseases of unknown cause might be caused by an infectious agent.

It may be that Tp is implicated in the aetiology of some cancers, particularly the lymphomas (classically Hodgkin's disease) and leukaemias. Obviously, pinpointing the links between infections and cancers poses a huge challenge for researchers, but it is recognised that infections can cause damage to human DNA and lead to changes within the cells. Doctors from Cancer Research UK made the claim that clusters of childhood cancer could have been caused by an unknown bacterium or virus following a study of 5000 cases of childhood cancer over 50 years, which indicated that an infection could strike a whole area at a time to cause leukaemia as well as brain and lymph cancer cases. (The findings were presented at the European Cancer Conference in Copenhagen.) At the same time, Public Health officials in Cornwall, UK, launched an investigation into a cluster of rare bone cancers that had killed 6 children near Penzance, and reported that "the obvious cause would be INFECTION". Other research, conducted decades ago, prompted banner headlines in newspapers asking "CAN YOU CATCH CANCER"!

CONCLUSIONS AND COMMENT

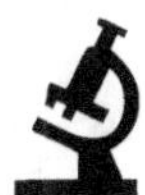

TRILLIONS OF DOLLARS, POUNDS, euros and yen of investment and decades of research into many of the major life-threatening diseases have failed to identify cause for any of them, and without known cause no treatment has been formulated to provide CURE. Decades of usage of armamentaria of ever more sophisticated drugs has only provided, at best, palliative or ameliorative relief or prophylactic cover and the diseases remain chronic, and morbidity and mortality high. Tens of millions of the global population are treated life-long with anti-coagulants, anti-hypertensives, anti-inflammatories, antibiotics, anti-ulcerants, anti-depressants, anti-asthmatics, etc., and not one of them has been provided with a cure for their disease. Many still suffer debilitating effects, some still die, because the PRIMARY cause of their disease has not been dealt with. Obviously, most diseases are highly complex and it could be argued that further investment and even more intensified research might eventually yield answers. Equally, if current research is on the wrong track (guided there by the Cabal, diversionary tactics and claims, and because the possibility of a single infectious cause is not thought credible) the answers might never be found. These revelations provide a different starting point and a different direction, and pencil in many explanations and solutions. Currently, world-wide, many groups of workers are engaged in researching particular disease areas. All are attempting to solve their particular puzzles. Some groups have found lots of pieces to their puzzle and can fit some of them together, whereas others have only a few pieces to their puzzle and cannot do anything with them. These revelations provide a picture of the much larger, completed puzzle and gives them the key piece (with plausible explanation) which they either did not have because of cover-ups, or they had left on the side. The theory of single cause uniquely satisfies the aetiological, pathological, immunological and epidemiological features and the pathogenesis of many chronic diseases – where cause is unknown and cure unachieved by conventional medicine – and offers an explanation of the inter-relationships and familial linkages apparently inherent for some of them. It also satisfies the historical picture. Recognition of Tp infection in the population, in developed communities specially, is only currently delimited by the wide held view that the infection is a sexually transmitted disease with a few well defined, easily identifiable clinical signs, which is easily diagnosed and picked up by screening programmes. That is known not to be the case – S, and its development, is a much more subtle disease. If all the known routes of transmission and clinical sequalae of the disease are acknowledged, and the fallibility of tests and testing procedure for the organism are admitted, then the disease becomes highly visible throughout the global population and the historical development of the disease is explained. Such theory also provides answer to the question of where a highly infectious widespread disease which has been around a long time and which is not self-limiting, has never been tackled head-on and which did not die out naturally, has gone to in an unprotected human population. Tp infection has always been, and remains, a threat to Humanity. S has been recognised in mass epidemics throughout history – in Europe from the 15th century onwards, in the Americas post Colombus, and in famed individuals from musicians to monarchs, poets to presidents, and now as frequent new outbreaks and epidemics of the infection occur on top of the background endemic situation. Such 'events' however are most often missed. Multi-symptom epidemics (any of a range of different symptoms such as headache, conjunctivitis, epigastric crisis, adenitis, sore throat and 'flu, etc., occurring in different individuals) would be difficult to recognise unless one of those symptoms predominated, when cause would probably be attributed to a common cause of such symptoms such as legionella, salmonella, mystery virus, etc., when bacteriological and epidemiological evidence to substantiate such diagnosis and conclusion is often, at best, very sparse and circumstantial. Many such epidemics lack a point source of contact and a causative organism cannot be isolated in the vast majority of individuals. Such epidemics are commonly much more widespread, with a wider range of clinical signs and degrees of severity of disease than is recognised or reported, and in many cases the overall infection pattern and clinical sequalae of such events better describes an observed outbreak of a bacterial infection. Examples in the UK would include an outbreak of an infectious respiratory order (supposedly Legionnaires disease) in Staffordshire in 1985 (reported in the Lancet, Jan '96) when patients admitted to hospital during the epidemic proved NOT to have the legionella bacterium and subsequent investigation found that the outbreak followed an epidemic of 'flu-like illness and some deaths in the surrounding community. Other examples in recent times would include epidemics seen in Wakefield, Liverpool and Cardiff mental hospitals, concurrent 'salmonella and scabies' epidemics in two girls' schools, a 'Legionella' outbreak centred on the BBC building, 'unseasonal' influenza outbreaks when 'flu virus was known not to be circulating, cluster meningitis in Stroud and elsewhere, and other multiple case medical events. Such events would represent only some observed points of a continually spreading disease which has many clinical manifestations and are well explained by the known transmissibility and early clinical signs of Tp infection.

Paradoxically it is probably in civilised populations – where transmission of Tp is presumed to be limited by good hygiene, sanitation, etc., and therefore where S is least expected to occur – that recognition of the disease in all its different guises is poorest, and where mis-diagnosis or the willingness to attribute an illness to an alternative but unknown cause is greatest. This hypothesis explains many medical events and the specific aetiological, pathological, immunological and epidemiological features of many diseases. It uniquely rationalises the progression of a disease through history and presents a picture of where that disease is now and could provide a new direction for the resolution of many diseases for the benefit of future generations. Such resolution would currently demand the distribution and administration of appropriate antibiotics life-long to the global population pending the development of an effective 'vaccine'. Without eradication of the bacterium, or until such strategy is employed however, many diseases will remain unresolved and Tp infection will continue, as it always has done, to ravage the planet. Reassuringly, it can be said that the world population is NOT suffering from syphilis – that is just one of many manifestations of Tp infection. Instead it should be said that the world is still, centuries on, exposed to a bacterial pandemic that has massive rates of mortality and morbidity. The current coronavirus pandemic illustrates the many reasons (socio-economic chaos, panic, lack of effective treatment, etc.) that were foreseen with a reveal of the treponemal pandemic and why it was covered up. As previously stated, Tp is a multi-system disease which has the potential to affect any organ in the body. The organism has become endemic in communities worldwide and may never go away. The world has unknowingly had to live with it for a long time, but there have been other lethal pathogens that the world has learned to live with (HIV, MERS-CoV, EBOLA, SARS-CoV, current SARS-CoV-2, and new pandemic 'flu viruses. Most of those diseases have continued as a threat because immune systems have not been primed to, or cannot, launch any defence against them, and no treatments have been formulated to eradicate them. Treponema pallidum continues as a threat because, despite its high rates of mortality and morbidity and the need for an effective treatment and global treatment programme, it was long ago deemed to be out of control and impossible to eradicate so its prevalence and the range of diseases it caused were covered up and the pandemic has been allowed to continue. The world has paid a high price for that cover-up.

The theme of this book – that **Tp IS THE SINGLE CAUSE OF MANY DISEASES** (and that the bacterium is transmitted in a continuous pandemic) - had been submitted for publication to a number of respected medical journals some time ago. Not unexpectantly, the hypothesis was rejected by all. It was obviously difficult to present a lateral, generalist view to specialists and the hypothesis challenged decades of medical doctrine, but none of the editing panels 'shot down' the premises or conclusions on which the theory was based. A common response was that it "did not fit the style of our journal"! Their rejection might also have been based on their thinking that the problem was irresolvable, alarmist to the populace, or a reveal of the collusion, conspiracy and cover-up by a Cabal of which they might be part. Such powerful parties have a vested interest in keeping such information from the general population. Fear of seriously de-stabilising the worlds of Medicine, Government, Industry, Finance etc., and causing panic and social and economic chaos within the global community (as observed in the throes of the current coronavirus pandemic and anticipated by the Tuskegee study team decades ago) was probably also a factor. The conclusions in this book hold for many medical arguments. In its entirety it offers solution and explanation to many medical unknowns, and a more rational argument and explanation than much current theory.

So, how is the world to be told something which it does not want to hear, or can do nothing about? How can one re-write the medical text-books, fight prejudice and jealousies, with claims that are tantamount to implying ignorance, incompetence or cover-up? Perhaps by alluding to the Truth! *The Rod of Asclepius* depicted on the front of this book has been widely adopted as the symbol for medicine and health but it has also been interpreted as representing **'a search for the truth amidst dark activity'**. The content of this book is exactly that! The symbol is usually interpreted as 'a serpent entwined around a staff' - a reasonable interpretation as the ancient Greeks used snakes as a panacea and *cure* for all ills. But could it be that the Greeks, long ago, suspected that a spiral organism rather than a serpent or snake *caused* all ills and that their god Apollo (father of Asclepius and god of 'healing, truth and *prophesy*') had prophesised such?

The terrible error of judgement and actions of the Cabal many years ago and through to this day, and the lack of action and capacity to deal with the pandemic and its sequalae, has meant that the world population has paid a very high price in terms of mortality and morbidity. To continue to not challenge that cover-up is tantamount to committing the same crime. As Plato is purported to have said "the price good men pay for indifference to public affairs is to be ruled by evil men". The Tuskeegee study researchers initially, and the members of the Cabal and their puppets later, with an admission of impotence and inability to do anything about the situation, denied future researchers the chance to find a solution. Had hygiene measures and social distancing (as practised today in the onslaught of the coronavirus pandemic) been introduced in an era of much reduced global connectivity, and decades of energetic research into the finding of an effective anti-spirochaetal agent been encouraged in the last 80 years, Tp infection might have been brought under control or even eradicated to benefit countless millions of the population and all future generations.

The revelations in this book will not be well received and the arguments and the conclusions will be met with hostility. It will be easy to dismiss this exposé as not true because that suits the World's narrative and the conclusions will upset the central dogma, but incredulous as these revelations are, such opposition does nothing to contradict those conclusions, and without challenge, the two contagions – the bacterium and the Cabal – will continue to deny the world population good health!

THE SPIRAL IN THE MAZE

REVEALING A COVER UP OF THE MOST LETHAL PANDEMIC IN HISTORY AND THE SINGLE CAUSE OF MANY DISEASES

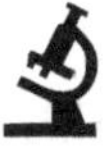

joanna phillips

LARGE PRINT

The Spiral in the Maze by Joanna Phillips

Contributors: Cover design and interior by AuthorPackages.com

ISBN: 9798657451689

Contents

"When hearing something unusual, do not pre-emptively reject it, for that would be folly. Indeed, horrible things may be true, and familiar and praised things may prove to be lies."

-Ibn Al-Nafis, 13th century physician and researcher who discovered cure for some diseases.

PANDEMICS

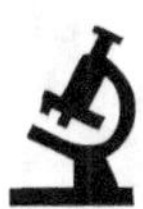

The greatest threat to human health - a contagium with rates of mortality and morbidity many times higher than any other patho-gen, ever circulating in a continuous pandemic – exists, but the identity of that threat has been covered- up, and death and many diseases have been attributed to 'other' or 'unknown' causes. Some perspective and the degree of threat posed by such a contagium can be realised by looking at the effects of past pandemics.

The 'Spanish' 'flu pandemic of 1918-19 infected an estimated 400 million people (a quarter of the then world population) and, with a mortality rate of about 15%, was responsible for the deaths of between 50 – 100 million. Small pox, with an estimated mortality rate of 30% killed an estimated 500 million in its existence. HIV / AIDS caused more than 36 million deaths at a peak rate of 2 million a year. The Asian 'flu pandemic of 1957-58 killed between 1 and 2 million people. SARS–CoV, causing Severe Acute Respiratory Syndrome in 2002–3, had a relatively high rate of mortality (10%) but only a low rate of infectivity so was only fatal to relatively few, and localized epidemics were contained by actions which slowed down or broke the chain of transmission. However, that virus was not eradicated and, with mutation, was forecast to cause a more lethal and widespread pandemic in the future. The current coronavirus (SARS–CoV–2) pan-demic, causing Covid–19, - with a very high rate of trans-mission and infectivity and a rela-tively low mortality rate (2-4%?) - has the potential to kill millions worldwide. If a significant percent-age of the world population is in-fected with a pathogen of only a moderate mortality rate, the total number of deaths would be high. It is interesting (and alarming) to compare the 'R' value (the spreada-bility factor or how many people are infected by a single carrier) of the 'Spanish' 'flu virus (R = 2.1) with that of the current coronavirus (pre-lock-down R = 2.5). That would seem to Indicate a pending global disaster. The R factor indicates the rate of infection in a pandemic and means that a contagium with a high value, even with a relatively low mortality rate, can result in a high number of infected individuals and cause panic and severe disruption of social and economic activity. In all the above epidemics and pandem-ics, the contagium is a virus, but there have also been pathogenic *bacterial* contagions which have proved fatal to many millions of the population. In the 14th century the 'Black Death' (caused by the bacterium Yersinia pestis) killed an estimated 75 – 200 million people worldwide. During the 20th century Mycobacterium tuberculosis caused 100 million deaths (half of those Infected). But there is one contagium which has rates of transmission, infectivity, mortality and morbidity many times higher than any of the contagions (viral or bacterial) mentioned above, the <u>continuing</u> presence of which HAS BEEN COVERED UP FOR DECADES. The presence of a long-time circulating pathogenic contagium was suspected more than three quarters of a century ago and a decision was made NOT to alert the populace. The realization that the cause of many deaths and diseases had been around for decades, even centuries, and could not be stopped or eradicated at that time (and even now), coupled with the thought that revealing the presence of such a threat to Humanity would cause panic and social and economic chaos, compelled the researchers to restrict their findings to as few people as possible. Thereafter, the collusion, conspiracy and cover-up must have involved members of the medical profession, editing boards of medical journals, governments, the pharmaceutical industry, and the media. Members of the Nobel Prize committee would join that Cabal later. It is plausible that the Hippocratic Oath – 2000 years old but amended many times according to changes in medicine, ethics, attitudes, etc. - has been amended to maintain a veil of secrecy over cover-ups. The more recent amendments promise: *"And whatsoever I shall see or hear in the cause of my profession, as well as outside my profession, in my intercourse with Men, if it be what should not be published abroad, I will never divulge – holding such things to be holy secrets"*. And: *"Whatever I may see or hear in the course of treatment in regard to the life of Man, which on no account one must spread abroad. I will keep to myself, holding such things shameful to be spoken about".* Because of the cover-up and an inability to *globally* treat and eradicate the Infectious agent (decades ago, and now) the contagium of the pandemic has continued to circulate round the globe, continuing to cause death and disease on a massive scale. Circulating for decades, even centuries, this contagium – a bacterium – has indiscriminately infected all age groups, regardless of ethnicity, geography, etc. In the womb, through life, that bacterium, a spirochaete, remains a sinister and unavoidable threat to BILLIONS of people on the planet. And it may have been suspected centuries ago! A quotation attributed to Desiderius Erasmus in 1520 says *"If I were asked which is the most destructive of all diseases, I should unhesitatingly reply it is that which for some years has been ravaging with impunity. What contagium does thus invade the whole body, so must resist medical art, becomes inoculated so readily, and so cruelly tortures the patient?"*. He asked the question against a background of a mysterious epidemic, hitherto unknown, which struck terror into all hearts by the rapidity of its spread, the ravages it made, and the apparent helplessness of physicians to cure it.

PROSPECTIVE STUDIES

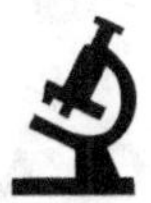

A number of studies have been conducted to observe the progress of untreated disease. Common among them for observation was the bacterium Treponema pallidum (Tp) - recognised as the causative organism of syphilis (S). In

1928, a Norwegian retrospective study carried out on several hundred white males, reported on the pathological manifestations of untreated syphilis. Four years later, an American study group decided to build on that Oslo work and perform a <u>prospective</u> study to complement it. [A prospective, observational study is normally employed to look at the long term sequalae of a known or suspected cause, or the effect of suspected risk factors that cannot be controlled. Such epidemiological studies, being observational in nature, examine the causes and development of disease in the human population. Cohorts of subjects are followed over time in longitudinal studies, the population of interest being monitored before, and when, particular disease-related outcomes occur. The studies watch for outcomes such as the development of a disease during the study period, and relate that to factors such as suspected cause or risk.] The American study, conducted between 1932 and 1972 in Tuskegee, Alabama by the US Public Health

Service became the infamous and unethical 'Study of untreated syphilis(S) in the negro male' - later to be cited as "arguably the most infamous biomedical research study in US history" and described by one researcher as "the economic exploitation of humans as a natural resource of a disease that could not be cultivated elsewhere, in order to establish and sustain US superiority in patented biotechnology". The Tuskegee Study, the purpose of which was supposedly to observe the natural history of untreated S, was carried out on 600 African-American men who were 'recruited' by being told that they were receiving free health care from the US Government. Two-thirds of the men had previously contracted S before the study began but none were told they had the disease. By 1947, Penicillin had become the standard treatment for (early) S in the general population (and other antibiotics were available in later years), so the doctors involved in the study had the chance of treating all their syphilitic subjects and closing the study, or splitting off a control group for testing with Penicillin . Instead, the Tuskegee researchers continued the study without treating any participants, with-holding the antibiotic and information about it from the men and preventing them from accessing S-treatment programmes in the surrounding areas. The study continued under the control of numerous US Public Health Service supervisors, including the Centre for Disease Control who, in the 1960s reaffirmed the need to continue the study. It ended in 1972 after 40 years of study, when a 'leak' to the media resulted in the trial's termination – the Washington Star, then the New York Times front page article, captured national attention and protest. By the end of the study most of the participants had died from the disease or related complications, 40 wives had been infected and 19 of their children were born with congenital S. The range of mortality and morbidity, and range of complications and disease observed in the 40 years of study, mirrored that of the general population, then and now.

The Tuskegee Study, in recognising the threat of Tp to individuals, also revealed the 'credentials' of Tp to be responsible for, and cause, many diseases as it's sequalae. However, that Tp was the single cause of many diseases of the Western world would also remain a secret – known only to the study team and the Cabal of medics, government officials, members of big pharma, and the media, that the team deigned to include in that knowledge. The scale and spread of the disease would, from that time, be masked by censorship. Scientific advisory groups around the world advise and guide governments on health emergencies, but their identity, 'credentials' and work, is shrouded in secrecy so it has always been difficult to challenge the decisions and recommendations being made. Governments do not publish member's names, or their medical or research backgrounds for 'security reasons' and thereby the anonymity of members of the Cabal is maintained.

In 1997, President Bill Clinton formally apologised on behalf of the

US, to victims of the experiment. The lack of ethical standards in the Study led to the establishment of the Office for Human Research Protections and new federal laws and regulations requiring Institutional Review Boards for the protection of human subjects in studies involving them, but the conclusions of the Study remained unreported. So why the notion and need for a non-treatment experiment? Probably because the researchers knew that S could not be treated on a global scale and eradicated, so needed to observe the natural progression of the disease to determine all of its sequalae.

Other studies had been conducted as the threat of Tp infection to the population was suspected or recognised. In a 1946-47 study in Guatemala, US researchers used prostitutes to infect prison inmates, insane asylum inmates and soldiers with S in order to test the effectiveness of Penicillin as treatment. People who had been infected with direct inoculations of preparations of Tp were also included in the trial. Approximately 700 people, including orphan children, were infected as part of the study which was sponsored by the Public Health Service, the National Institute of Health and the Pan-American Health Sanitary Bureau (now part of The World Health Organization). The American leader of the team had chosen to do the study in Guatemala because he would not have been permitted to conduct it in the US. He later participated in the Tuskegee Experiment.

THE THEORY OF SINGLE CAUSE

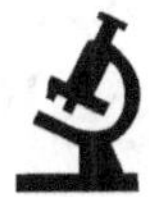

The suspicion that a treponeme, as the primary cause of massive mortality and morbidity in the world, carried on a continuously circulating global pandemic and causing many of the major chronic diseases of the human population, is further strengthened by a number of sum-mary premises:

- ⚗ Tp is a highly infectious bac-terium transmissible by virtu-ally every route.

- ⚗ Tp is not a self-limiting infec-tion, nor is it susceptible to the body's defence mecha-nisms.

- ⚗ Tp has been globally wide-spread for centuries.

- ⚗ A global programme to eradi-cate the bacterium has never been implemented.

Given those 4 premises, Tp MUST have spread, and be still spreading, virtually unchecked, resulting in frequent epidemics and global pandemic which will have left the disease endemic in many countries.

Further:

- ⚗ Tp is known to cause all the clinical sequalae characteristic of many chronic diseases.

- ⚗ Recognition of S – particularly it's secondary and later manifestations – is difficult.

- ⚗ Screening for S is limited and

the sensitivity of tests for Tp is questionable.

⚗ Administration of anti-Tp antibiotics in high dose, extended course regimens has been very limited, so that most of the global population remains untreated for Tp infection.

The indication is therefore, that many diseases are the result of a single cause – infection by the same contagium (Tp) - which, as main primary cause, satisfies the aetiological, pathological, immunological and epidemiological features and patho-genesis of many diseases. To accept that indication – that a specific disease is caused by a specific organism – the organism should satisfy the basic scientific requirements of 'The Postulates of Koch', which states that:

- The micro-organism must be found in abundance in all subjects suffering from the disease, but should not be found in healthy people.

- The micro-organism must be isolated from a diseased host

and grown in pure culture medium.

⚗ The cultured micro-organism should cause disease when introduced into a healthy sub-ject.

⚗ The micro-organism must be re-isolated from the inocu-lated, diseased, experimental host and identified as being identical to the original, spe-cific, causative agent.

Apart from the inherent limitations that could not be resolved in the late 19th century, and the subtlety and denial of Tp causing many diseases, those postulates do not account for 'agents' that cannot be grown in culture media. Whilst many bacterial pathogens of humans satisfy Koch's postulates, Tp cannot be grown in cell-free culture media, as is also the case for Helicobacter pylori (see later as supposed cause of duodenal ulcer) and the leprosy causing bacterium. They, similarly, do not fulfil all of Koch's postulates.

As previously stated, epidemiologists refer to the *Reproduction Number* (R) which is the number of new infections an infectious person would be able to generate. (common 'flu has a value of 7; measles ca.15). The R number for Tp infection would be very high based on the duration of time that a person is infectious, the opportunities that person has to spread the organism whilst infectious, the probability that with transmission at least one of those opportunities results in infection, and the average susceptibility of the population to that infection. According to that epidemiologists' formula, a very high R value would indicate that the contagium cannot be contained. That established widespread disease and its cause could not be stopped from spreading would have been recognised in the Tuskegee Study.

At any time, without limitation or eradication, the contagium would continue to infect the global population. Tp is highly transmissible by virtually every route but primarily by physical contact, salival transfer, ingestion, and aerosol transmission (the aerosolisation of the bacterium from normal breathing). Sexual transmission of the organism is incidental to the main spread of the disease. Resulting disease, as apparently wide-ranging as Coronary Heart Disease, Sudden Infant Death Syndrome, Multiple Sclerosis, Myalgic Encephalomyelitis (chronic fatigue syndrome), Peptic Ulcer disease, Dementia (and other neurological diseases), Diabetes, Arthritis and others, are <u>different manifestations of the same disease.</u>

A single cause of those diseases would explain many of the specific pathological, immunological and epidemiological features of many diseases, and the links, inter-relationships and commonly observed associations between many of them, and suggests that vertical transmission of Tp rather than genetic inheritance is the explanation of familial traits for some diseases, and that vertical and horizontal transmission of the organism dictates time of onset and spread pattern of many of those diseases. Natural attenuation (especially during vertical transmission of a disease), change, increased host tolerance and the widespread use of antibiotics for unrelated(?) condi-tions, has probably resulted in forms of Tp and manifestations of its dis-eases which do not fit the older, classical forms and descriptions of those diseases, making recognition and diagnosis of a disease even more difficult. The effectiveness of sensitivity tests for Tp and current screening procedure is doubted.

Whilst an individual in the early stages of Tp infection can suppos-edly be cleared of the contagium, and the development of a disease prevented, by administration of a

course of an antibiotic (e.g. penicillin), the difficulty in eradicating the
highly transmissible pathogen from
the global population is obvious, especially as successfully(?) treated
individuals are vulnerable to (re)in-
fection the minute they step back
into the community. Recognition of
those facts was probably the reason
for the Tuskegee Study. Tp has a
very high R number and, with current global connectivity facilitating
even greater transmission possibilities, means that at that level the
contagium cannot be contained. The

Tuskegee Study group realised that the Tp pandemic was already out of control in the 1940s! Also, just as age, ethnicity, geography and climate have no influence on the distribution of Tp, neither do they affect the intrinsic transmissibility or infectivity of the organism. At best it can be said that social habit (hygiene, dress, isolation) might reduce the opportunities for transmission, but the potential for transmission of the organism by multiple routes in any population – where Tp is anyway known to be circulating (= endemic) - must remain high. S has been globally widespread for centuries and until recently was recognised as one of the most common and important diseases in the world. The oldest known case from which Tp has been isolated was the mummified remains of a 16th century socialite, and the disease was known to be very common by that time. S was first recognised in epidemic form in Europe, and in the Americas post Columbus, in the 15th century, and in the Renaissance Period was known as the Neapolitan disease.

Since then, the problems of aetiology and treatment have engaged the attention of many investigators but the fundamental contributions to present knowledge were all made before 1910! The causal organism was identified in 1905 (Schaudinn and Hoffman); a test was developed in 1906 (Wassermann); and a treatment (arsenic) introduced in 1910 (Ehrlick). Early writings going back to Hippocrates make reference to a disease which was probably S. The disease even warranted a poem by Frascatorius in 1530 and a mention in Shakespeare.

Tp is not a self-limiting infection and is not susceptible to the body's defence mechanisms, as evidenced by the fact that the disease can manifest itself many decades after initial infection. The serious clinical sequalae of the infection develop very slowly and insidiously. A mechanism capable of destroying the treponemes in the blood and tissues during secondary S is not known. (It is not phagocytosis as the treponemes seem able to resist engulfment by leucocytes, and lytic processes involving complement and specific antibody have not been identified). Without specific treatment the disease develops and causes a wide range of serious clinical sequalae. The Oslo and Tuskegee Studies were devised to determine the course of untreated S, and from those and other studies it was commonly thought that about 10% of those infected and untreated develop cardiovascular lesions, 10% neurological lesions, and 15% lesions in other tissues, and that 65% of patients with untreated S did not develop late sequalae of the disease – a strange assumption considering the clinical severity of disease in the other 35%! The evidence suggests that the range of clinical sequalae of untreated S is much wider and encompasses many other diseases and degrees of disease. S is a highly infectious disease especially in its early stages, commonly recognised as the first 2 years. Although S is recognised as a sexually transmitted disease, it is known to be transmissible by virtually every other route and non-venereal S is known. It has been supposed that in developed communities especially, transmission was limited because the disease was thought to be spread almost exclusively by sexual intercourse and little opportunity presented for it to be spread by other forms of direct contact under normal conditions of social life. However, it is known that the source of infection can be extra-genital and in non-venereal S rapid transmission of the delicate treponemes occurs – particularly by mouth. All lesions of primary and secondary S – especially those involving the mucous membranes (for which Tp has a particular predilection) on exposed surfaces – discharge very large numbers of treponemes and constitute large reservoirs of infection and a very great hazard. Such lesions may remain infective for as long as 4-5 years until they heal. Other common extragenital sites known include the lips, tongue, mouth, tonsils, pharynx, eye-lids, fingers, hands and any part of the skin and mucous membranes. Infection has been reported in lesions on the hands of medical and nursing staff dealing with cases of S. Further, endemic non-venereal S is known and is common in some countries. It is known that the treponeme responsible for causing *venereal S* and *endemic non-venereal S* is the same – it is morphologically, immunologically, and serologically IDENTICAL. The two diseases are differentiated only by definition based on considerations of climate, geography, age of onset and route of transmission. Venereal S is acknowledged to have global distribution without climatic, geographic, racial or age barriers, whereas non-venereal S has been subjectively delimited to a childhood disease with limited geographical distribution. Such an age definition would automatically exclude any later manifestations of the disease (involvement of vascular tissues, organs, CNS, etc.) some decades later. The fact that endemic non-venereal S (caused by Tp) exists and can affect 60% of some childhood populations confirms the absolute transmissibility and infectivity of the organism via extra-genital sites. That potential for transmission and infectivity must exist globally. The general incidence, spread and development of untreated S, and the range, degree and subtlety of the disease is much greater than has been traditionally thought because the facts and the observations in the long-term prospective studies have been covered up, so for those 'experts' outside the Cabal, the disease has spread unrecognised, unchecked and mis-diagnosed. A coordinated global programme to eradicate Tp infection has never been implemented. The disease is acknowledged to have been globally widespread for centuries and by the afore-mentioned premises must have continued to spread. An effective treatment for an individual has only been available, or applied, in the last 80 years, and previous epidemics must have left a massive reservoir of untreated, infected (and infectious) individuals. *Recognised* early infectious S reached its peak just after the second world war and the advent of penicillin supposedly made a dramatic and rapid impact on that incidence of disease. Early WHO-or-chestrated programmes in parts of Africa, the Middle East and Yugosla-via had limited success, but for a variety of reasons (socio-economic, competing medical priorities, health administrators over-impressed by early success, etc.) such pro-grammes were not properly consoli-dated, nor further continued, nor expanded into other areas, so that relapse and re-infection resulted. Treatment of whole communities in a national, international or global progamme to eradicate the disease has never been undertaken. That must have left the vast majority of the world population untreated, to constitute a large reservoir of infection with massive potential for continued transmission, so the disease would remain endemic in some countries and a global pandemic would continue. The continuing high prevalence of S in developing countries, and the 'resurgence' of the disease in advanced countries was recognised and noted by the WHO more than 40 years ago.

Although antibiotics have since

been widely used for a range of infections, relatively few individuals will have received an appropriate antibiotic in high enough dosage administered at the right time or for long enough time to eradicate Tp so spread of the disease in all infected populations must have continued. Even those few individuals successfully(?) treated would be liable to re-infection as continuous interface, interaction and traffic at family, community, national and international level would facilitate continuous spread of the disease, unless a global policy of effective treatment of the population was undertaken. The risk of an outbreak of S from an individual presenting with classic symptoms of the disease and the threat of Tp infection to any population *is* currently recognised and guarded against. However, current screening policy – that employed in routine diagnosis and mass screening programmes – is heavily reliant on tests designed to indicate disease *activity.* Such tests often react negatively in late or latent disease and will fail to indicate the extent of vertically acquired disease or disease contracted horizontally early in life. What has not been recognised nor guarded against by those outside the Cabal is the absolute transmissibility of the bacterium, the less than classic and wide range of symptoms of later disease and the risk to the global population – factors which demand a coordinated treatment policy on a global scale. Those factors have been covered up (with an admission that an effective treatment was not available for a global population and the pandemic has

long been out of control?), so without such a policy the disease has
spread, and will continue to spread
throughout the global population. It
is worth noting that the current and
earlier coronavirus infections
achieved global distribution in
months, and the AIDS virus - with
limited routes of transmission and a
relatively low rate of infectivity - in
less than two decades. By contrast,
the potential of an infectious agent
which has been around for centuries, is transmissible by virtually all
known routes, and has never been

'challenged' globally, must be un-limited. WHO acknowledges 40 million new cases of S being notified worldwide annually. That must be the 'tip of the iceberg'. With the possible exception of small isolated communities, Tp infection must be currently endemic in most countries, and in a continuing pandemic, billions of the world's population must have been infected.

Treponema pallidum is KNOWN to cause all the clinical sequalae shown by, and characteristic of, the major chronic diseases. WHO's '*Interna-*

tional Classification of Diseases' devotes more pages to, and attributes more clinical sequalae to syphilis than any other disease. It is known that Tp can affect virtually every tissue, organ and system of the body and can cause most conditions and mimic most 'other' diseases. The clinical signs of disease attributed to Tp infection are clinically indistinguishable from the clinical signs attributed to supposed other causes. For example, the signs of cardiovascular disease attributed to Tp are no different from those of aortic incompetence and aneurysms from 'other' causes. S has always been known as the most subtle of all diseases and thought a master of disguise. There is no symptom that it cannot cause, and no syndrome for which it may be responsible. Virtually every disease in part has been attributed to Tp infection. Research, as in the Tuskegee Study and others, suggests that Tp infection is the MAIN cause of those diseases.

Recognition of the disease at any stage is difficult. Any of the stages of the disease can be absent or so inapparent as to be overlooked, and a diagnosis of S from its secondary and later clinical signs would be unlikely. Primary infection with Tp and first clinical signs of S ('flu-like illness, adenitis, etc.,) are often missed, and without that recognition subsequent clinical manifestations of the disease many years later (coronary heart disease, dementia, etc.) will be most unlikely to be diagnosed as S or be associated with that disease. S is a general systemic infection in the course of which certain lesions are produced in different tissues which may be sufficiently striking to attract medical attention. Without recognition of the primary disease, those lesions will almost certainly be labelled 'other disease'. Such manifestations of S will most often be mis-diagnosed. As a result, most such patients will never be tested for S, have their condition di-agnosed as S, or be treated for S. As an illustration, a patient presenting with later manifestations of the dis-ease – such as damage to the cardi-ovascular system with destruction of elastic tissue and formation of aneurysms in the large arteries - would (without recognition of the primary phase) be diagnosed *only* as having coronary heart disease. Recognition of Tp infection in the clinical situation is extremely poor. The Tuskegee Study showed that the incidence of sub-clinical disease (especially cardio-vascular lesions and aortitis) was at least twice as high as clinically diagnosed disease, and there is evidence that patients with S are more prone to 'other' diseases.

Screening for Tp infection in the

population is limited. The bacterium is hard to find and identify, and the sensitivity of tests for it is questionable and further compromised by many factors. Essentially, to be diagnosed positive for Tp infection depends on when and how an individual is tested. Confirmation of Tp infection, and diagnosis of S, even for the few showing classical primary clinical signs (as in those with venereal S) is extremely difficult, and standard tests for S - the tests most likely to be employed in general screening procedures - are not sufficiently specific or sensitive for complete diagnostic reliability and results can also be compromised by other factors. It is known that in primary S, none of the tests available is 100% conclusive, even if conducted at the right time relative to the time of initial infection, and ALL serological tests can be negative despite the presence of a primary lesion. Further tests are supposedly more specific but would normally only be carried out if initial screening results were positive and are, anyway, compromised by a number of factors. It is known that the available tests can be variously compromised by lack of specificity; lack of serological reactivity of the bacterium (which may be due to a capsular or slime layer sometimes observed on the surface of Tp); scarcity of treponemes (as in very early, latent and late stages of the disease); slow or non-appearance of antibody (reagin) in serum; excess reagin normally produced in some patients; and antibiotic usage (even months before). All those factors would induce a negative reaction to the tests. Positive reactions can be similarly misleading and can be caused by many (other) microbial infections and pathological lesions (which can liberate lipid antigens in the tissues and consequently form lipoidophil antibodies on which some tests are based). Supposed false positive reactions are frequently seen in blood donors, pregnant women, and those with an infection, but are usually attributed to other factors, or contradicted by further tests. Infections such as glandular fever, mumps, chicken pox, herpes simplex, herpes zoster and viral(?) pneumonia can cause positive results to a test many months after the infection, and rheumatoid arthritis and many auto-immune diseases (disseminated lupus erythematosus, haemolytic anaemia, thyroiditis, etc.) can cause positive reactions to those tests for many years, even a life-time. The fact that rheumatoid arthritis, many supposed auto-immune diseases, microbial infection, and unconfirmed glandular fever and mumps show positive to standard tests for S would seem to con-

firm the presence of Tp. It is suggested that many of the supposed
false positive reactions are in fact a
true positive reaction to Treponema
pallidum. The fact that the KNOWN
incidence of false positive and false
negative results in those tested is
high, must question the effectiveness of the screen for Tp – a screen
which anyway is reserved for a very
small percentage of patients selected from genito-urinary departments, ante-natal clinics, transplant
centres, blood transfusion centres
and some neurological wards. The

sensitivity of available tests and even the premise on which some of them are based (eg: antibody production) is questionable. The presence of Tp, at whatever stage in the progression of the disease, is extremely difficult to determine even by trained analysts, but an inability by Science to show the presence of Tp does not mean that it is not present, or has not been present, as the causative organism of a particular disease. It is known that in Tabes Dorsalis for example (an extreme and advanced form of S) Tp is NOT found in the tissues. Like many bacterial infections the chronicity of the inflammatory reaction is often inversely proportional to the number of organisms seen, and that phenomenon is apparent in the many diseases caused by Tp. In late or latent cases of syphilis ALL tests (even the more specific tests) can be negative, and a high percentage (>20%) of late cases react negatively to the standard tests for S. Also, the fact that even after supposedly adequate treatment with appropriate antibiotics, the VDRL test can remain positive for some time, and the FTA and TPHA tests often remain positive for life. That must seriously question the sensitivity of the tests, or the effectiveness of treatment, or both, or invite the conclusion that Tp is present and that those tests are showing true positives. It must be remembered anyway, that the vast majority of patients suffering secondary and later manifestations of S (such as cardiovascular disease, dementia, MS, arthritis, etc.) will never have been suspected of having S so will not have been subjected to those tests. Being in older age groups with long-standing disease, they would probably test negatively anyway. Even with such limitations, random screening of an aged population will show >2.5% of them to have Tp infection and in those tested for the infection the number of confirmed infected individuals is greatly underestimated. The effectiveness of testing is therefore doubted and supportive claims for the effectiveness of the tests have not enough basis to deflect anything from these facts.

Administration of antibiotics which are active against Tp and which are given at high enough dosage or for long enough time to eradicate the organism is very limited. Unless a patient is being treated specifically for confirmed S, most antibiotics – employed empirically to treat other infections – are unlikely to be given in a regimen effective enough to eradicate Tp, even if the bacterium was included in its spectrum of anti-bacterial activity. That means that for most of the global population and despite the widespread use of antibiotics, without recognition and cor-rect diagnosis of the primary dis-ease, the secondary and later mani-festations of the disease will be un-treated, under-treated or mis-treated.

Procaine penicillin (by injection) remains the treatment of choice for all types of (confirmed) S and suc-cessful treatment depends on achieving high blood and tissue con-centrations and maintaining those over at least two weeks. 100% cure rates are unknown, and cure rates for other antibiotics in the treatment of S (e.g. oral erythromycin, tetra-cyclines, cephalosporins) are signif-icantly lower even when used at the required levels, and in empirical use for other infections would be most unlikely to effect clinical cure and eradication of the bacterium. The ef-fectiveness of antibiotic therapy is difficult to determine. Tp is suppos-edly extremely sensitive to penicillin and during treatment healing of le-sions occurs and the treponemes disappear from early stage lesions. Biological cure however (= complete eradication of the treponemes) is difficult to prove since the bacterium cannot be cultured in vitro. It is known that in some patients who have been 'adequately' treated with procaine penicillin, residual treponemes have been detected in cerebro-spinal fluid and lymph nodes. Those bacteria have not acquired resistance to the antibiotic because surviving treponemes, after inoculation into rabbits, produce typical lesions where they are penicillin sensitive. It may be then that the treponemes migrate to less accessible tissues, such as neural and skeletal tissue, where levels of antibiotic are not sufficiently high to effect complete eradication of that bacterial population so that reservoirs of treponemes remain in those tissues. The potential for a large number of infected individuals to remain in any population, even after treatment, therefore must be significant.

The prognosis for treated S depends on the stage of the disease and the degree of tissue damage that has occurred in vascular, neurological and other systems. Whilst successful treatment may result in

clinical cure and stop the inflammatory process and progression of disease, the tissue damage may have
been too great to prevent an improvement in symptoms and the
disease would be regarded as
chronic.

The widespread use of antibiotics
for unrelated(?) conditions has
probably resulted in forms of Tp and
manifestations of S which do not fit
the older, classical, clinical definitions, which must confuse further
the clinical picture and make diagnosis even more difficult. As

previously said, such antibiotics, in empirical use, are unlikely to be given in high enough dose or for long enough to eradicate Tp even if they are active against the bacterium. The most widely used antibiotic in the UK – amoxycillin – is not active against Tp in normal dosage regimens. It is interesting to note that in the US and Japan - where cephalosporin antibiotics have been used extensively for the past 20 years - the incidence of coronary heart disease has coincidentally declined. Cephalexin for example is active against Tp if given as high dose, extended courses. It may be then, that the widespread use of certain antibiotics may have had some effect in limiting the progression of Tp infection, but the incidence of late manifestations of the infection would remain high. Such an observation would indicate that a globally implemented antibiotic programme might have some success and benefit future generations, but implementing such a programme would not be possible in practical terms. That was recognised by the Tuskegee Study team and was the reason for the Study.

PATHOLOGY AND PATHOGENESIS

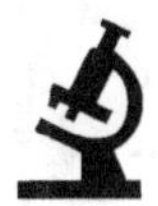

In looking at the pathology and pathogenesis of Tp infection, it is suggested that infection by that bacterium – achieved by virtually any route of transmission to any of a number of sites (mainly mucous membranes of the nasopharynx, mouth and digestive tract) – results in the first clinical signs of penetration such as chancre and ulcer of the mouth, stomach or duodenum. Where the infection occurs 'in utero' (Tp can cross the placental barrier), conditions such as hole in the heart and cleft lip and palate may result. Tp is a spirochaete (a spiral organism), superbly designed for penetration into even intact tissue and capable of boring, corkscrew and thrusting movements. (Also, it is now known that the bacterium is micro-aerophilic rather than a strict anaerobe – a property which facilitates transfer outside the body.) After penetrating tissue, the treponemes invade the perivascular lymph spaces where they multiply rapidly and massively to excite the syphilitic reaction. That consists of an accumulation of mononuclear cells (lymphocytes and monocytes) to form a focus of inflammatory tissue which is highly vascular. Fibroblasts are stimulated to proliferate and 'healing' occurs with replacement of inflammatory cells by fibrous tissue. The degree of fibrosis and the type of host tissue would determine the visibility of the initial chancre or ulcer which can be very discreet, especially in thin mucous membranes. Such lesions, and any serum that exudes from them, contain very large numbers of treponemes and all lesions of secondary S – especially those involving mucous membranes on exposed surfaces – discharge very large numbers of treponemes. As such they constitute large reservoirs of infective material for transmission and a very great hazard. Such lesions may remain infective for as long as 4-5 years, until they heal. A site in the mouth therefore would have a potential for infecting others (by aerosol droplet or salival transfer) and might facilitate a direct route to the central nervous system via the mucous membranes and the sinuses.

Before the first lesion has appeared (commonly 10 – 90 days after initial infection) the treponemes undergo massive multiplication (with a generation time of less than

5 hours are capable of producing billions of organisms in days) and infect the entire body. Initially the treponemes invade the lymph nodes where they cause an adenitis, and from the regional lymphatics are rapidly conveyed to the blood stream in large numbers, and from there to the various tissues. The adenitis at this stage would most likely be diagnosed as 'viral infection', 'glandular fever' or 'mumps' and as such would not be treated. A common clinical sign of Tp infection at this stage is a 'flu-like illness, often

severe and of protracted length, which usually occurs within 3 months of initial infection. Tp has a known predilection for mucous membranes and the fact that 'respiratory infection', a 'cold' or 'snuffles' is a common pre-cursor to infant cot death (which commonly occurs around 3 months of age) strongly implicates Tp and infection in the first few days / weeks of life, as the primary cause of Sudden Infant Death Syndrome. A 'flu-like reaction to Tp infection is only one of a number of known initial clinical signs. Other indications of such infection include headaches, swollen glands, rashes, general malaise, iritis and conjunctivitis, gastritis, weight loss, and meningitis. In the very young, the elderly, sick or immuno-compromised, this first manifestation of Tp infection may be fatal. Occasionally, patients can suffer recurring 'first manifestations' with recurrent bouts of colds, 'flu, and throat and respiratory tract infections. Glandular fever or 'recurrent infection' would commonly be diagnosed. After such clinical sequalae which, without notice of a primary syphilitic reaction, would be mis-diagnosed and therefore untreated or mis-treated, the disease can enter a period of quiescence during which time the foci of infection can remain dormant and undetected in the tissues for a long time. Alternatively, the disease develops insidiously to cause later serious clinical sequalae, but whereas early clinical manifestations of S are probably due to the vast numbers of treponemes and their effects, later manifestations of the disease are probably the result of delayed hypersensitivity and inflammatory reactions to the products or toxins of the bacterium and the presence of relatively few persisting treponemes. Like other chronic bacterial infections (e.g. tuberculosis) chronicity of the inflammatory reaction is often inversely proportional to the number of organisms seen, and lesions of tertiary S contain very few treponemes. Over a long period, certainly years, sometimes decades, it is thought that Tp causes a general demyelination of fatty tissues - a destruction of fats and muco-proteins - or an interference with their metabolism, causing breakdown of elastic tissue, extensive tissue damage and exposure of nerve fibres. Such effect may be mediated by immune complexes. A principal pathological effect of Tp infection is damage to the cardiovascular system with destruction of elastic tissue and the formation of aneurysms in the large arteries. Tp is believed to spread to the aorta during the early stages of the infection, possibly via the lymphatics and the mediastinal nodes.

The treponemes lodge in the aortic wall and may remain dormant for years. The eventual consequence is destruction of the muscular and elastic layers of the aortic wall and replacement with functionally inert scar tissue. Sudden unexpected death is frequently associated with aortic regurgitation and angina. It is estimated that in those patients with cardiovascular lesions, 30% died as a direct result of it, and lesions of cardiovascular S are not infrequently found at autopsy in selected populations as a chance finding. It has also been observed that simple syphilitic aortitis has been diagnosed in 5 – 10% of people during life.

In the smaller arteries and capillaries, at a more discreet level or earlier in the process, such effect may cause general hypertension or, in the heart, coronary insufficiency. Hyperlipidaemia and atherosclerosis may be the result of deposition of degraded fatty materials leached from tissues, or a compensatory response by the body to make up the 'loss' caused by the effects of Tp infection. Changes in fat composition have also been observed in the liver of victims of SIDS, and in peptic ulcer disease mucous loss is noticeable at the site of ulceration.

In the lung, disease of the small pulmonary arteries would cause pulmonary hypertension with associated symptoms and sequalae. In the brain, the degree of narrowing of the arteries might variously cause headaches, migraine, neuroses, psychoses, epilepsy and dementia before any cerebral atrophy or thrombosis is identified. In Diabetes, carbohydrate and fat metabolism is disordered and the defect leads to the appearance of atherosclerosis early in patients with that disease. Atherosclerosis itself may be a compensatory response by the body (working on negative feedback instruction) to make up the 'loss' caused by Tp.

It has been established that many patients with rheumatoid arthritis die from infections and renal diseases, and in some studies an increased mortality from cardiovascular, gastro-intestinal and respiratory diseases was reported. A reported excess of deaths from malignancies in patients with rheumatoid arthritis remains controversial.

Damage to the CNS remains sub-clinical for a long time – often several decades – but at an extreme would include destruction of the fatty coating around nerve fibres. In some CNS disorders it is known that an accumulation of amyloid precursor protein (APP) causes impairment of axonal transport with deposition of amyloid and plaque formation, and recent studies have shown that axon degeneration precedes and sometimes causes neural death. Dying back processes may underlie early loss of synapses that occurs in Alzheimers disease for example. Other CNS disorders with APP positive axon pathology include the acute demyelinating diseases such as Parkinsonism, MS, Motor Neuron Disease, Creutzfeldt-Jakob disease, senile dementia and HIV dementia. In Alzheimers, MND and Parkinsonism, damage to specific regions of the CNS leaves the affected areas especially prone to the consequences of neuronal attrition. Tp should be considered as one of the 'triggers' and cause of axon death in many disorders.

Different symptoms of the disease are probably a result of the different tissues developing hypersensitivity to Tp and its products and reacting differently to the irritation with different inflammatory responses and degrees of response. The fat and muco-protein loss results in an overall 'drying out' and loss of lubrication and elasticity in the affected tissue which can then become hypersensitive to irritants and liable to dysfunction. Such reaction is classically seen in asthma, hay fever and skin disease such as eczema, which are often related. A greater and chronic inflammatory response is observed in lupus erythematosus and arthritis. Other principal pathological effects include the formation of chronic granulomata in skin, bone, the internal organs and the brain. A dose response relationship would be expected for neuronal damage of infectious origin and there could be considerable interindividual variation in susceptibility. Trace of the causative organism is often gone long before the appearance of those diseases.

Evidence of a direct link between chronic sinusitis and MS (by spread of infection from a diseased sinus into the CNS) once prompted examination of an old 'spirochaetal hypothesis' which has been shown to be not erroneous, and a spirochaetal infection of the CNS would explain the specific pathological, immunological and epidemiological features of MS.

The degree of association between Schizophrenia and organic disease exceeds that expected by chance and it is thought that in some cases the organic disease is of major aetiological importance. The most common organic states associated with Schizophrenia are epilepsy, neurosyphilis, alcohol and drug abuse, and those common associations cannot be dismissed as chance findings as they occur too often in the presentation and course of schizophrenic illness to be ignored. Those observations suggest that most such supposed age-related neuronal attrition is a consequence of demyelination of nerve tissue due to infection by Tp. It is therefore suggested that demyelination is mediated by immune complexes as a result of infection with Tp and that **TREPONEMA PALLIDUM IS THE PRIMARY CAUSE OF A NUMBER OF DISEASES.**

RANGE OF DISEASE

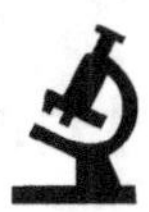

Tp infection is ubiquitous and largely sub-clinical for many years. The initial infection might take place before birth or in very early life although the disease may not appear until much later. The infection can be passed through sperm or the ovum and be transmitted trans-placentally, perinatally or postnatally through close contact. The body's inability to deal with the bacterium would then allow the development of future disease. The diseases include those of the vascular tissues - heart attack, stroke, hypertension, atherosclerosis and hypercholesteraemia and 'cluster meningitis'; diseases of the CNS such as senile and familial transmissible dementia, motor neuron disease, Parkinson's disease and Alzheimer's disease; obstructive airways disease, asthma and recurrent 'bronchitis'; rheumatoid and osteo-arthritis; ME; skin disease including eczema, psoriasis and varicose ulcers; multiple sclerosis; duodenal and gastric ulcer disease; Crohns disease; Sudden Infant Death Syndrome and 'in utero' events such as cleft lip, cleft palate (the world's 3rd most common birth defect), hole in the heart, still-birth and spontaneous abortion. In SIDS, the finding of unusually high levels of immunoglobins in the lungs of cot death babies lends weight to the theory that death results from an anaphylactic reaction to a respiratory infection.

Victims of the syndrome often have an upper respiratory tract infection in the week before death so the pathogen would have stimulated or disrupted the immunoglobin production system and exposed the infant to a full attack from the bacterium. Reyes Syndrome is an acute childhood illness with vomiting and coma that typically occurs a few days after a mild infection and the pathogenesis is usually attributed to generalized mitochondrial dysfunction caused by a bacterial, viral or toxic agent in a genetically susceptible host. Crohns disease and ulcerative colitis are ten times more common in immediate family members of patients with those diseases compared with the general population. A link between a bacterium and Crohns disease has not been clearly established but controlled trials have shown that long-term treatment with an antibiotic (metronidazole, effective against anaerobes) can be effective in both colonic and perianal Crohns disease. Investigations to determine whether an infectious agent is involved in the aetiology of

Crohns suggest that because the occurrence of the disease in married couples is greater than that expected by chance, spouses of patients might be at particular risk of contracting the disease, which supports the view that an infectious agent might be involved. Most of those diseases are KNOWN as late manifestations of Tp infection and catalogued as such in the WHO 'Classification of Diseases'. It is worth noting that 'an infectious agent' or 'unknown virus *infection*' is often proposed in the aetiology of many of those diseases. Newspaper headlines many years ago posed the question "is infection the cause of a heart disease epidemic?"

Recognising Tp as the primary cause of many diseases also explains the commonly observed associations, links and inter-relationships of many supposed 'distinct' diseases. Such associations are known between asthma and eczema, hypertension and obstructive airways disease, diabetes and skin disease, retinopathy and blindness, osteomyelitis and cutaneous chronic ulcers, sinusitis and MS, and sexually transmitted disease and 'juvenile' arthritis. Also, as an objective overview, this hypothesis unifies many diseases which are currently only differentiated by subjective interpretation, description and name. Similarly, it offers an alternative explanation to genetic inheritance for some diseases. Vertical transmission of Tp would account for familial traits seen in coronary heart disease, hypertension, atherosclerosis, hypercholesteraemia, asthma, eczema, ulcerative colitis, Crohns disease and some dementias. Early, juvenile and late onset forms of many diseases would be a result of the time of initial Infection with Tp relative to either vertical or horizontal transmission of the organism - as where traditional adult diseases occur in children (stroke in infants; heart attack in juveniles). The organism can cross the placental barrier and can be transmitted to the foetus throughout pregnancy. The degree of maternal disease *activity* probably dictates the time of onset and severity of disease in pregnancy, so that the effect may range from extreme and immediate (intra-uterine or neonatal death) through congenital disease in the infant or child, to more subtly manifest disease many years later in the adult. Second and third generation S is known. Vertically acquired infection may also render the individual refractory to subsequent horizontal infection. Additional support for this thinking comes from the fact that treponemes have actually been identified in association with some diseases (peptic ulcer disease and multiple sclerosis) and postulated as the cause of MS via the sinuses. In the early 1900s several reputable neuropathologists noted the similarity of the clinical and histological characteristics of MS and neurosyphilis, and reported the presence of treponemes in the plaques of Multiple Sclerosis. **The theory that Multiple Sclerosis was caused by a treponeme has never been disproved.**

In the light of this hypothesis Tp should also be considered as the primary cause of Guillain-Barre disease, Creutzfeldt – Jacob disease, Reiter's syndrome, Henloch-Schlonlein purpura, Gertsmann – Straussler syndrome, Erythema Infectiosum (5th Disease), Occult Subacute Thyroiditis. And Cancer? - Tp might be implicated in the aetiology of lymphomas (Hodgkin's Disease) and leukaemias (see later).

This hypothesis may also offer an explanation for the development of full-blown AIDS after HIV infection. It is thought that other factors besides the virus are needed for a substantial lowering of T4 cell levels and progression to full blown AIDS. Tp itself can profoundly depress T4 cell levels and may be an important con-tributor or co-factor. Seroconversion studies have suggested that sex-ually transmitted co—factors, pre-seroconversion and/or post-sero-conversion, play a role in the pro-gression of HIV infection. The effect may simply be additive when the rate of progression from HIV infec-tion to full-blown AIDS would be dic-tated by the degree of syphilitic ac-tivity in the presence of the virus. Fastest actual decline could be anticipated if Tp infection or early active disease occurred at the time of HIV infection or sometime post-seroconversion (Tp acting on the viral genes that regulate HIV expression in the host cell); slowest decline could be anticipated if the virus infection occurred on top of a late or latent syphilitic state, or if Tp was not present. Where latent S exists, destruction of the immune system by HIV might allow development of a disease in the same way as latent TB develops when 'unmasked' by the virus. Alternatively, HIV might act purely opportunistically in a Tp compromised host, or similarly Tp in an HIV compromised host. Widespread incidence of Tp infection would explain the ultimate high conversion rate of HIV infection into full-blown AIDS. In all those scenarios, appropriate antibiotic treatment and long-term prophylaxis might mean HIV infection not progressing to full-blown AIDS.

DIVERSIONARY MEASURES

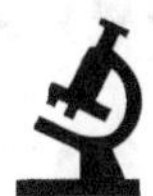

There have been many outbreaks of disease which could be attributed to Tp as the cause, and some diseases and cause appear to have been deliberately covered up, viz: The Tuskegee study and Helicobacter pylori causing ulcers study.

In the early 1980s a physician at the University of Western Australia, set out to show that the bacterium Helicobacter pylori (Hp) played a major role in causing peptic ulcer disease, challenging decades of medical doctrine holding that ulcers were caused primarily by stress, spicy foods, excess acid, etc., and instead adopted the theory that peptic ulcers were caused by a bacterium – an idea first postulated 150 years ago (Bottcher and Letulle, 1875). The presence of bacteria-like organisms in the lumen of the gastric glands was also noted by Klebs in 1881, and Jaworski in 1889 described spiral organisms in sediment washings of humans and suggested those organisms might be involved in gastric ulcer disease. A century ago, different researchers found spirochaetes in the stomachs of mice, cats, dogs and cows, and in the early 20th century a number of researchers found spirochaetes associated with peptic ulcer disease. In 1936, the first edition of the Russian 'Large Medical Encyclopaedia' suggested infection was one of the causes of peptic ulcer disease. In 1939 Friedberg found Hp in the human stomach but abandoned his research after his boss advised him to move to another subject! Hp was generally regarded as a harmless commensal organism in the stomachs of millions of people. In the 1950s a number of researchers (Allende, in 1951, Tarnopolskaya in 1955, Gordon in 1958) used penicillin to treat gastric ulcers, and since then numerous researchers found bacteria associated with peptic ulcer disease. Their reported findings were often rejected for publication.

In 1982 the researchers in Australia began their first study to determine the relationship between Hp and peptic ulcer disease (PUD) The letters referencing that research were published in the Lancet in 1983. A year later, one of the research team intentionally consumed a large inoculum of Hp and became ill (as would be expected with the ingestion of any bacterial culture!) He then self-medicated with antibiotics and was relieved of his symptoms and those observations were published in 1985. **INGESTING THE CULTURE OF Hp DID NOT IN-DUCE AN ULCER.** Ingestion of Hp has been shown to cause gastritis in many animal subjects but has NEVER been shown to induce ulcer formation. The claim that eradication of the bacterium (in this case Hp) with antibiotics and substantially reducing the occurrence of ulcers would equally apply to any bacterium (including Tp which has better 'credentials' for causing ulcers). Hp is linked aetiologically to histological GASTRITIS but a pathogenic role for Hp in duodenal ulcer (DU) disease is unproven and whilst Hp might fulfil Koch's postulates for histological GASTRITIS, it does not fulfil them for DUODENAL ULCERATION. Studies suggest that eradication of Hp infection is associated with a significant reduction in the relapse rate of DU, independent of other factors. In patients remaining culture negative for one year, both histological gastritis and DU recurrence were unlikely. That does not prove that Hp is of aetiological importance in DU disease. Hp has been implicated in the pathogenesis of gastritis, DUs, GUs and even gastric cancer but ASSOCIATON and CAUSE should not be confused. Hp is a bacterium which characteristically grows attached to gastric epithelial cells and is commonly found in the gobal population with easy transmission (orally or by ingestion), usually within families. That makes it an ideal 'fall-guy' to divert attention from other possible causes. It was observed that patients with recurrence of Hp infection tended to experience relapse of their DU disease, whereas those in whom complete eradication had been achieved were much less likely to have a recurrence of duodenal ulceration. That would be the case if another bacterium was the causal organism. Examination of the distribution of peptic ulcer sites has revealed that they occur most commonly on either side of the pyloric sphincter. In the stomach, ulceration of the gastric mucosa occurs in the narrowed part of the stomach where transition of Tp from a contaminated bolus of food and penetration into the near-by gastric wall would be relatively easy, and a gastric ulcer would result. After exit through the pylorus, a contaminated bolus would immediately enter the narrowest section of the duodenum and the bacterium would be close to the duodenal mucosa with opportunity for transmission from the food bolus and perforation of the duodenal wall to cause a duodenal ulcer.

Evidence that infection precedes the first ulcer is difficult to prove because endoscopy is rarely done in people without symptoms. In DU relapse however, recurrence of Hp infection after apparent eradication is probably due to the original strain surviving antibiotic treatment (indicating failure of eradication), re-infection with Hp or a less sensitive causative bacterium. Pharmaceutical company promotional literature to doctors at that time showed that recurrence of Hp after treating the ulcer with antibiotics was very low. The literature did not show recurrence rates of PUD. An extensive study in Dublin demonstrated that eradication of Hp with antibiotics substantially reduced the re-occurrence of ulcers, but that would also be the result if the antibiotics were eradicating a different causative bacterium. Ingestion of Hp has been shown to cause gastritis in many animal studies (and by the researcher himself!) but has NEVER been shown to induce an ulcer. Nowhere has Hp been shown to be the cause of peptic ulcers; the evidence is only circumstantial. As previously stated, Hp fulfils Koch's postulates for histological gastritis but does not fulfil them for duodenal ulceration, but the researchers' claims got antibiotics used for ulcer treatment, and the recommended regimens would be effective against treponemal infection and true cause. The lead researcher was awarded the Nobel Prize in 2005. But for what? The formulation of a new cocktail? Hp broth as a new gastronomic treat? Certainly not for identifying the cause of PUD. That award questions the gullibility, integrity or involvement with the Cabal of those Stockholm and Frankfurt committees and the committee awarding the Ehrlich and

Darmstaedter prize in 1977. The research was continued in the US where the process was required to be accelerated - which ultimately the National Institute of Health and the FDA did by fast-tracking a lot of the existing 'knowledge' into the US, and getting others to conduct repeat studies to *confirm* the results and 'get the news out' (1990s). A conference held by the NIH(USA) demonstrated the general acceptance in the US of Hp as the cause of PUD. The medical community had been finally convinced; the cover-up had been consolidated. Despite the conclusions and claims for Hp, the lead researcher still conceded that an infectious cause for most diseases that remain unexplained could not be ruled out.

CANCER

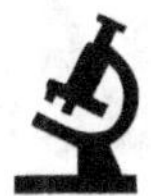

The researcher also claimed that Hp was the cause of stomach cancer. He had observed that everybody who got stomach cancer developed it on a background of gastritis, and in patients without Hp, gastritis was not evident. He concluded that because the only important cause of gastritis was Hp (according to him), therefore that bacterium had to be the most important cause of stomach cancer as well!! Treponema pallidum would be a better candidate as the causal agent for stomach cancer (and for other cancers as well). As previously stated, that researcher had conceded that many diseases of unknown cause might be caused by an infectious agent.

It may be that Tp is implicated in the aetiology of some cancers, particularly the lymphomas (classically Hodgkin's disease) and leukaemias. Obviously, pinpointing the links between infections and cancers poses a huge challenge for researchers, but it is recognised that infections can cause damage to human DNA and lead to changes within the cells. Doctors from Cancer Research UK made the claim that clusters of childhood cancer could have been caused by an unknown bacterium or virus following a study of 5000 cases of childhood cancer over 50 years, which indicated that an infection could strike a whole area at a time to cause leukaemia as well as brain and lymph cancer cases. (The findings were presented at the European Cancer Conference in Copenhagen.) At the same time, Public Health officials in Cornwall, UK, launched an investigation into a cluster of rare bone cancers that had killed 6 children near Penzance, and reported that "the obvious cause would be INFECTION". Other research, conducted decades ago, prompted banner headlines in newspapers asking "CAN YOU CATCH CANCER"!

CONCLUSIONS AND COMMENT

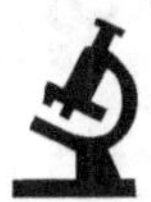

Trillions of dollars, pounds, euros and yen of investment and decades of research into many of the major life-threatening diseases have failed to identify cause for any of them, and without known cause no treatment has been formulated to provide CURE. Decades of usage of armamentaria of ever more sophisticated drugs has only provided, at best, palliative or ameliorative relief or prophylactic cover and the diseases remain chronic, and morbidity and mortality high. Tens of millions of the global population are treated life-long with anti-coagulants, anti-hypertensives, anti-inflammatories, antibiotics, anti-ulcerants, anti-depressants, anti-asthmatics, etc., and not one of them has been provided with a cure for their disease. Many still suffer debilitating effects, some still die, because the PRIMARY cause of their disease has not been dealt with. Obviously, most diseases are highly complex and it could be argued that further investment and even more intensified research might eventually yield answers. Equally, if current research is on the wrong track (guided there by the Cabal, diversionary tactics and claims, and because the possibility of a single infectious cause is not thought credible) the answers might never be found. These revelations provide a different starting point and a different direction, and pencil in many explanations and solutions. Currently, world-wide, many groups of workers are engaged in research-ing particular disease areas. All are attempting to solve their particular puzzles. Some groups have found lots of pieces to their puzzle and can fit some of them together, whereas others have only a few pieces to their puzzle and cannot do anything with them. These revelations pro-vide a picture of the much larger, completed puzzle and gives them the key piece (with plausible explanation) which they either did not have because of cover-ups, or they had left on the side. The theory of single cause uniquely satisfies the aetiological, pathological, immuno-logical and epidemiological features and the pathogenesis of many chronic diseases – where cause is unknown and cure unachieved by conventional medicine – and offers an explanation of the inter-relation-ships and familial linkages appar-ently inherent for some of them. It also satisfies the historical picture. Recognition of Tp infection in the population, in developed communities specially, is only currently delimited by the wide held view that the infection is a sexually transmitted disease with a few well defined, easily identifiable clinical signs, which is easily diagnosed and picked up by screening programmes. That is known not to be the case – S, and its development, is a much more subtle disease. If all the known routes of transmission and clinical sequalae of the disease are acknowledged, and the fallibility of tests and testing procedure for the organism are admitted, then the disease becomes highly visible throughout the global population and the historical development of the disease is explained. Such theory also provides answer to the question of where a highly infectious widespread disease which has been around a long time and which is not self-limiting, has never been tackled head-on and which did not die out naturally, has gone to in an unprotected human population. Tp infection has always been, and remains, a threat to Humanity. S has been recognised in mass epidemics throughout history – in Europe from the 15th century onwards, in the Americas post Colombus, and in famed individuals from musicians to monarchs, poets to presidents, and now as frequent new outbreaks and epidemics of the infection occur on top of the background endemic situation. Such 'events' however are most often missed. Multi-symptom epidemics (any of a range of different symptoms such as headache, conjunctivitis, epigastric crisis, adenitis, sore throat and 'flu, etc., occurring in different individuals) would be difficult to recognise unless one of those symptoms predominated, when cause would probably be attributed to a common cause of such symptoms such as legionella, salmonella, mystery virus, etc., when bacteriological and epidemiological evidence to substantiate such diagnosis and conclusion is often, at best, very sparse and circumstantial. Many such epidemics lack a point source of contact and a causative organism cannot be isolated in the vast majority of individuals.

Such epidemics are commonly much more widespread, with a wider range of clinical signs and degrees of severity of disease than is recognised or reported, and in many cases the overall infection pattern and clinical sequalae of such events better describes an observed outbreak of a bacterial infection. Examples in the UK would include an outbreak of an infectious respiratory order (supposedly Legionnaires disease) in Staffordshire in 1985 (reported in the Lancet, Jan '96) when patients admitted to hospital during the epidemic proved NOT to have the legionella bacterium and subsequent investigation found that the outbreak followed an epidemic of 'flu-like illness and some deaths in the surrounding community. Other examples in recent times would include epidemics seen in Wakefield, Liverpool and Cardiff mental hospitals, concurrent 'salmonella and scabies' epidemics in two girls' schools, a 'Legionella' outbreak centred on the BBC building, 'unseasonal' influenza outbreaks when 'flu virus was known not to be circulating, cluster meningitis in Stroud and elsewhere, and other multiple case medical events. Such events would represent only some observed points of a continually spreading disease which has many clinical manifestations and are well explained by the known transmissibility and early clinical signs of Tp infection.

Paradoxically it is probably in civilised populations – where transmission of Tp is presumed to be limited by good hygiene, sanitation, etc., and therefore where S is least expected to occur – that recognition of the disease in all its different guises is poorest, and where mis-diagnosis or the willingness to attribute an illness to an alternative but unknown cause is greatest. This hypothesis explains many medical events and the specific aetiological, pathological, immunological and epidemiological features of many diseases. It uniquely rationalises the progression of a disease through history and presents a picture of where that disease is now and could provide a new direction for the resolution of many diseases for the benefit of future generations. Such resolution would currently demand the distribution and administration of appropriate antibiotics life-long to the global population pending the development of an effective 'vaccine'. Without eradication of the bacterium, or until such strategy is employed however, many diseases will remain unresolved and Tp infection will continue, as it always has done, to ravage the planet. Reassuringly, it can be said that the world population is NOT suffering from syphilis – that is just one of many manifestations of

Tp infection. Instead it should be said that the world is still, centuries on, exposed to a bacterial pandemic that has massive rates of mortality and morbidity. The current coronavirus pandemic illustrates the many reasons (socio-economic chaos, panic, lack of effective treatment, etc.) that were foreseen with a reveal of the treponemal pandemic and why it was covered up. As previously stated, Tp is a multi-system disease which has the potential to affect any organ in the body. The organism has become endemic in communities worldwide and may never go away. The world has unknowingly had to live with it for a long time, but there have been other lethal pathogens that the world has learned to live with (HIV, MERS-CoV, EBOLA, SARS-CoV, current SARS-CoV-2, and new pandemic 'flu viruses. Most of those diseases have continued as a threat because immune systems have not been primed to, or cannot, launch any defence against them, and no treatments have been formulated to eradicate them. Treponema pallidum continues as a threat because, despite its high rates of mortality and morbidity and the need for an effective treatment and global treatment programme, it was long ago deemed to be out of control and impossible to eradicate so its prevalence and the range of diseases it caused were covered up and the pandemic has been allowed to continue. The world has paid a high price for that cover-up.

The theme of this book – that **Tp IS THE SINGLE CAUSE OF MANY DISEASES** (and that the bacterium is transmitted in a continuous pandemic) - had been submitted for publication to a number of respected medical journals some time ago. Not unexpectantly, the hypothesis was rejected by all. It was obviously difficult to present a lateral, generalist view to specialists and the hypothesis challenged decades of medical doctrine, but none of the editing panels 'shot down' the premises or conclusions on which the theory was based. A common response was that it "did not fit the style of our journal"! Their rejection might also have been based on their thinking that the problem was irresolvable, alarmist to the populace, or a reveal of the collusion, conspiracy and cover-up by a Cabal of which they might be part. Such powerful parties have a vested interest in keeping such information from the general population. Fear of seriously de-stabilising the worlds of Medicine, Government, Industry, Finance etc., and causing panic and social and economic chaos within the global community (as observed in the throes of the current coronavirus pandemic and anticipated by the Tuskegee study team decades ago) was probably also a factor. The conclusions in this book hold for many medical arguments. In its entirety it offers solution and explanation to many medical unknowns, and a more rational argument and explanation than much current theory.

So, how is the world to be told something which it does not want to hear, or can do nothing about? How can one re-write the medical textbooks, fight prejudice and jealousies, with claims that are tantamount to implying ignorance, incompetence or cover-up? Perhaps by alluding to the Truth! *The Rod of Asclepius* depicted on the front of this book has been widely adopted as the symbol for medicine and health but it has also been interpreted as representing **'a search for the truth amidst dark activity'**. The content of this book is exactly that! The symbol is usually interpreted as 'a serpent entwined around a staff' - a reasonable interpretation as the ancient Greeks used snakes as a panacea and *cure* for all ills. But could it be that the Greeks, long ago, suspected that a spiral organism rather than a serpent or snake *caused* all ills and that their god Apollo (father of Asclepius and god of 'healing, truth and *prophesy*') had prophesised such?

The terrible error of judgement and actions of the Cabal many years ago and through to this day, and the lack of action and capacity to deal with the pandemic and its sequalae, has meant that the world population has paid a very high price in terms of mortality and morbidity. To continue to not challenge that cover-up is tantamount to committing the same crime. As Plato is purported to have said "the price good men pay for indifference to public affairs is to be ruled by evil men". The Tuskee-gee study researchers initially, and the members of the Cabal and their puppets later, with an admission of impotence and inability to do any-thing about the situation, denied fu-ture researchers the chance to find a solution. Had hygiene measures and social distancing (as practised today in the onslaught of the coronavirus pandemic) been introduced in an era of much reduced global connectivity, and decades of energetic research into the finding of an effective anti-spirochaetal agent been encouraged in the last 80 years, Tp infection might have been brought under control or even eradicated to benefit countless millions of the population and all future generations.

The revelations in this book will not be well received and the arguments and the conclusions will be met with hostility. It will be easy to dismiss this exposé as not true be-cause that suits the World's narra-tive and the conclusions will upset the central dogma, but incredulous as these revelations are, such oppo-sition does nothing to contradict those conclusions, and without chal-lenge, the two contagions – the bac-terium and the Cabal – will continue to deny the world population good health!